MIMESIS
INTERNATIONAL

ATMOSPHERIC SPACES
n. 11

ATMOSPHERIC SPACES

Director: Tonino Griffero (*Tor Vergata University – Rome*)
Coordinator: Marco Tedeschini (*Tor Vergata University – Rome*)
Executive Secretary: Sara Borriello, Serena Massimo (*Tor Vergata University – Rome*)

Committee Members:

Niels Albertsen (*Aarhus School of Architecture*), Jean-François Augoyard (*CNRS – Grenoble*), Bruce Bégout (*Bordeaux Montaigne University*), Arnold Berleant (*Emeritus – Long Island University*), Mikkel Bille (*Roskilde University*), Gernot Böhme († *IPPh – Darmstadt*), Christian Borch (*Copenhagen Business School*), Gabor Csepregi (*University of Saint-Boniface – Winnipeg*), Christoph Demmerling (*Friedrich Schiller University – Jena*), Gianni Francesetti (*IPsiG – Turin*), Thomas Fuchs (*Heidelberg University Hospital*), Michael Großheim (*Rostock University*), Robert Gugutzer (*Goethe University – Frankfurt*), Hans Ulrich Gumbrecht (*Stanford University*), Jürgen Hasse (*Goethe University – Frankfurt*), Michael Hauskeller (*University of Liverpool*), Timothy Ingold (*University of Aberdeen*), Christian Julmi (*University of Hagen*), Rainer Kazig (*CNRS – Grenoble*), Robert J. Kozljanic (*Albunea Verlag – Munich; Nietzsche-Forum – Munich*), Hilge Landweer (*Free University of Berlin*), David Le Breton (*University of Strasbourg*), Juhani Pallasmaa (*Aalto University*), Alberto Pérez-Gómez (*McGill University – Montreal, Quebec*), Andreas Philippopoulos-Mihalopoulos (*University of Westminster – London*), Hermann Schmitz († *Emeritus – Kiel University*), David Seamon (*Kansas State University*), Giovanni Stanghellini (*Gabriele d'Annunzio University – Chieti; Diego Portales University – Santiago*), Shanti Sumartojo (*Monash University*), Jean-Paul Thibaud (*CNRS – Grenoble*)

Associate Members:

Aurosa Alison (*Polytechnic University of Milan*), Valeria Bizzari (*Catholic University of Leuven*), Guenda Bernegger (*SUPSI – Switzerland*), Alessandro Bertinetto (*University of Turin*), Margit Brunner (*University of Adelaide*), Elisabetta Canepa (*University of Genoa; Kansas State University*), Barbara Carnevali (*EHESS – Paris*), Vincenzo Costa (*Vita-Salute San Raffaele University – Milan*), Federico De Matteis (*University of L'Aquila*), Elisabetta Di Stefano (*University of Palermo*), Mădălina Diaconu (*University of Vienna*), Carsten Friberg (*Independent Researcher – Copenhagen*), Mildred Galland-Szymkowiak (*CNRS – École Normale Supérieure – Paris*), Julian Hanich (*University of Groningen*), Dehlia Hannah (*Arizona State University*), Klaske M. Havik (*Delft University of Technology*), Christiane Heibach (*FHNW Basel; University of Regensburg*), Maximilian Gregor Hepach (*University of Cambridge*), Yuho Hisayama (*Kobe University*), George Home-Cook (*Independent Researcher – UK*), Veronica Iubei (*Heidelberg University*), Steffen Kluck (*Rostock University*), Reinhardt Knodt (*Independent Researcher – Berlin*), Joel Krueger (*University of Exeter*), Wendelin Küpers (*Karlshochschule – Karlsruhe*), Rita Messori (*University of Parma*), Eugenio Morello (*Polytechnic University of Milan*), Werner Müller-Pelzer (*Fachhochschule – Dortmund*), Irina Oznobikhina (*European University – St. Petersburg*), Barbara Piga (*Polytechnic University of Milan*), Matthew Pritchard (*University of Leeds*), Tiziana Proietti (*Oklahoma University*), Andreas Rauh (*University of Würzburg*), Friedlind Riedel (*Bauhaus University – Weimar*), Simon Runkel (*Friedrich Schiller University – Jena*), Susanne Schmitt (*Independent Researcher – Munich*), Sara Asu Schroer (*University of Oslo*), Renata Scognamiglio (*Sapienza University – Rome*), Antonio Somaini (*Sorbonne Nouvelle University – Paris 3*), Anette Stenslund (*Roskilde University*), Thomas Szanto (*University of Copenhagen*), Juha Torvinen (*University of Helsinki*), Dylan Trigg (*University of Vienna*), Silvia Vizzardelli (*University of Calabria*), Izabela Wieczorek (*University of Reading*), Barbara Wolf (*Kolping Hochschule – Cologne*), Penelope Woods (*Queen Mary University – London*)

What is an "Atmosphere"?

According to an aesthetic, phenomenological and ontological view, such a notion can be understood as a sensorial and affective quality widespread in space. It is the particular tone that determines the way one experiences her surroundings.

Air, ambiance, aura, climate, environment, genius loci, milieu, mood, numinous, lived space, Stimmung, but also Umwelt, ki, aida, Zwischen, in-between – all these words are names hiding, in fact, the founding idea of atmospheres: a vague ens or power, without visible and discrete boundaries, which we find around us and, resonating in our lived body, even involves us.

Studying atmospheres means, thus, a parte subjecti, to analyse (above all) the range of unintentional or involuntary experiences and, in particular, those experiences which emotionally "tonalise" our everyday life. A parte objecti, it means however to learn how atmospheres are intentionally (e.g. artistically, politically, socially, etc.) produced and how we can critically evaluate them, thus avoiding being easily manipulated by such feelings.

Atmospheric Spaces is a new book series whose aim is to become a point of reference for a community that works together on this philosophical and transdisciplinary subject and for all those whose research, more broadly, is involved in the so-called "affective turn" of the Social Sciences and Humanities.

Elisabetta Canepa

ARCHITECTURE IS ATMOSPHERE

Notes on Empathy, Emotions, Body, Brain, and Space

Foreword by Tenna Doktor Olsen Tvedebrink

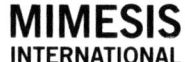

Translation: Sophie Henderson
Copy editing: Mikaela Wynne
Cover: Francesca Ióvene

© 2022 – MIMESIS INTERNATIONAL
www.mimesisinternational.com
e-mail: info@mimesisinternational.com

Book series: *Atmospheric Spaces*, n. 11

Isbn: 9788869773785

© MIM Edizioni Srl
P.I. C.F. 02419370301

CONTENTS

FOREWORD 9
Tenna Doktor Olsen Tvedebrink

PREMISE 11

I. A DEFINITION LACKING DEFINITION 15
  1. Rooms and Atmospheres 15
  2. Blurred Certainties 18
  3. A Challenge to the Vague 21
  4. Atmospheric Code 24
    First unknown: invisibility 24
    Second unknown: incorporeality 26
    Third unknown: uncontrollability 27
    Fourth unknown: complexity 28
    Fifth unknown: mutability 30
    Sixth unknown: subjectivity 32
    Seventh unknown: immaturity 33
    Eighth unknown: allusiveness 35
  5. Atmospheric Phenomenographies 37
  6. Seeds 40

II. ROOTS 43
  1. Semantic Geography 43
  2. Genesis 44
  3. Metaphorical Inversion 47
  4. Detonation 50
  5. Architectural Genealogy 52
  6. Thesaurus 56
  7. Coagulation 58

III. ATLAS OF ATMOSPHERES 61
  1. Network 61

2. Nodes 63
    First node: atmosphere as microclimate 63
    Second node: atmosphere as meteorological staging 67
    Third node: atmosphere as aesthetic-decorative quality 73
    Fourth node: atmosphere as the identity of a place 76
    Fifth node: atmosphere as collective imagination 81
    Sixth node: atmosphere as metaphor 84
    Seventh node: atmosphere as constitutive character 87
    Eighth node: atmosphere as aura 92
    Ninth node: atmosphere as collector of memories 94
    Tenth node: atmosphere as perceptive experience 98
    Eleventh node: atmosphere as mood 102
3. Interweaving 105

IV. ATMOSPHERIC REVIVAL 107
  1. Evolutionary Background 107
  2. Atmospheric Turn 109
  3. In Praise of Atmospheres 114

V. TO PERCEIVE THE INVISIBLE 117
  1. Experiencing Architecture 117
  2. Paradigm Shift 121
  3. Scientific Grounding 123
  4. The Polyphony of the Senses 126
    First property: atmosphere is composite 127
    Second property: atmosphere is unfocused 131
    Third property: atmosphere is multisensory 132
    Fourth property: atmosphere is multimodal 134
    Fifth property: atmosphere is kinaesthetic and haptic 134
    Sixth property: atmosphere is instinctive 137
  5. Atmospheric Bodies 138
  6. The Swarm of Emotions 143
  7. Empathic Contagion 150
    Empathy and architecture 150
    Visuomotor resonance mechanisms 156
    Embodied simulation 160

IN A NUTSHELL 165

BIBLIOGRAPHY 167

TENNA DOKTOR OLSEN TVEDEBRINK
FOREWORD

Atmosphere.
It is a poetic and vibrant word. An intriguing term. It is omnipresent. Universally recognised, it is an integral part of everyday vocabulary.

Yet atmosphere is a concept many students of architecture, design, and building engineering regard rather complex and difficult to grasp, discuss, and implement in their design processes. As an academic researcher and university teacher, I often hear complaints that the notion is too intangible, unstable, and subjective. Students find it nearly impossible to identify and measure. They struggle with translating it into concrete terms at the different design phases. Even some academic colleagues consider it a vague expression, which explains why it is frequently ignored or downplayed in both teaching and research.

With this book, Elisabetta Canepa continues a central theme in the literature on architectural theory, namely, understanding and debating the essence of atmosphere in architectural thinking. In this way, she builds on the work of Peter Zumthor, Juhani Pallasmaa, Gernot Böhme, Tonino Griffero, Alberto Pérez-Gómez, Harry Francis Mallgrave, and Sarah Robinson; not to mention that of Steen Eiler Rasmussen.

Departing from these architectural theoreticians, Canepa re-contextualises the question of atmosphere. She achieves this using an original and rigorous scientific approach, with the twofold aim of overcoming the vague character that the topic currently suffers from and comprehending the deeper meaning and functioning mechanisms of the term.

With the fascinating title *Architecture is Atmosphere*, Canepa emphasises the interesting point that a building is not merely an aesthetic object to visually adore, or a functional container to spatially optimize and occupy.

Rather, architecture *is* atmosphere — a phenomenon the human body perceives and empathise with on an emotional level. In other words, she highlights the importance of perception and sensory stimuli — and places lived experience and emotions at the fore.

In that sense, Canepa focuses attention on phenomenology and embodiment paradigm, in particular, incorporating elements of (neuro) biology and cognition — how human emotions, brains, and minds engage with the built environment —, to expand existing architectural theoretical frameworks.

In the last few years, the field of architecture has become increasingly attuned to the rapid developments in neuroscience and cognitive science. Of noteworthy interest is how technological and digital breakthroughs have made it possible to explore and test the human body and human experiences. These recent research achievements offer a series of innovative insights into architectural thinking. Canepa acknowledges these scientific implications and applies them to scrutinize the potential and limits of the topic of atmosphere. Her book provides, on the one hand, a significant introduction to and overview of the architectural literature debating the concept of atmosphere — from the early writings of Gottfried Semper and the later ones of Aldo Rossi and Christian Norberg-Schulz, to the more contemporary work of Tim Ingold. On the other hand, it is an exciting exploration of a new theoretical framework, outlined by five overall stages: *definition, evolution, mapping, revival,* and *scientific grounding.*

In summary, this volume helps clarify and categorise the notion of atmosphere in architecture. Furthermore, it aids to navigate the vast amount of literature (and design pathways) that exist on the topic. I admire Elisabetta Canepa for embarking on such a difficult journey, and I heartily recommend her work to all those who seek advice on the experiential qualities of architecture.

This book stands out to me as being a future key reference in architectural teaching and research on atmosphere. It is pertinent for both the novice student and the more experienced scholar.

Tenna Doktor Olsen Tvedebrink, PhD
Professor of Architecture, CREATE, Aalborg University
December 2021

PREMISE

When we enter a room, we become aware of the atmosphere.

Every contact with the vibrant sensoriality of a place generates atmospheric epiphanies — more or less intense, more or less engaging, and more or less intelligible — that resound with the personal sensibility of the individual. It is there, we suppose, the release of empathic symbiosis with the space in which we are immersed occurs. It is there that the experiential vocation of architecture takes form. It is there that the nebulous dimension of architectural atmospheres gets embodied, namely the dimension of the ineffable and ephemeral par excellence, what is impalpable and emotional, subjective and barely hinted. A condition that is apparently indeterminable, elusive, and without possible definition. To attempt to understand the meaning and functioning mechanisms of the atmospheric resource in the architectural field is the aim of this book.

Encroaching on other disciplines, such as aesthetics, phenomenology, and cognitive science, leads to striking out in new directions to find help in unravelling the enigma of atmosphere in architecture. The core, around which this journey through the maze of architectural poetics gravitates, seeking the expressive qualities of the built space,[1] is the *body* — root

---

[1] This book is a development of the author's doctoral research (Canepa 2019). The thesis *Neurocosmi: La dimensione atmosferica tra architettura e neuroscienze* ("Neurocosmos: The Atmospheric Dimension between Architecture and Neuroscience") was defended in May 2019 at the Department of Architecture and Design (dAD) of the Polytechnic School of Genoa, under the supervision of Valter Scelsi (architect and professor of architectural and urban design at dAD) and Anna Fassio (professor of human physiology and neurophysiology at DIMES — Department of Experimental Medicine, School of Medicine, University of Genoa). To conduct the final experiment, she also sought the collaboration of Laura Avanzino, neurologist and professor of neurophysiology, and Giovanna Lagravinese, psychologist and researcher — both belonging to DIMES.

and threshold of lived experiences. The exploration follows the steps dictated by a prototypical compass, intentionally assembled to navigate vagueness. Since it seems hard to glimpse a way through atmospheric vagueness, the philosopher Tonino Griffero, to whom we will often ask advice on this expedition, urges us — at least — "to stay in it in the right way" (2014a, 7).

As the German philosopher Karsten Harries (b. 1937) observes, "the need for building cannot be reduced to the need to achieve physical control of the environment" (1983, 16). Indeed, architecture, or rather the art and science of manipulating our surroundings, "produces atmospheres in everything it creates" (1991, 36), states Gernot Böhme (1937–2022), who shares Harries' nationality, profession, and year of birth.

It does, of course, solve objective problems and build objects, buildings of all descriptions. But architecture is aesthetic work inasmuch as rooms and space are always created with a specific quality of mood and hence as atmospheres. (Böhme 1991, 36)

Architecture is a complex process of spatial organisation, which is conceived, developed, felt, and communicated also (and above all) by means of its atmospheric manifestations. To tackle the nuanced and fleeting nature of the atmospheric event,[2] I have proposed registering a semantic definition, with which to formalise such an intrinsically vague notion, up to now hatched from architectural knowledge for the most part through metaphors and "ineffable"[3] expressions. Almost by paradox, I

---

2   See the first four chapters of the book. Chapter I "A Definition Lacking Definition" introduces the atmospheric issue within the architectural discipline, analysing its elusive essence: atmosphere is a complex phenomenon because it is invisible, intangible, without physical limits, multifaceted, unstable, highly subjective, often depicted by way of allusion, and still not structured in a recognised and shared architectural theory. — Chapter II "Roots" reconstructs the genealogy, evolution, and semantic network of the word "atmosphere," with particular attention to the architectural domain. — Chapter III "Atlas of Atmospheres" outlines a map to collect the miscellany of interpretations and uses of the atmospheric concept forged by the architectural culture over time. — Chapter IV "Atmospheric Revival" sheds light on the current phase of atmospheric stirring that inflames architecture, emphasising the urgency of finding a clear understanding of the atmospheric topic in the architectural context.

3   The reference is to the locution "ineffable space," coined by Le Corbusier (1948).

have synthesised a formula that follows *scientific criteria*.[4] Atmosphere becomes a describable and even potentially measurable entity — that can be submitted to assessment by experimental protocols (Canepa et al. 2019).

---

4   See chapter V "To Perceive the Invisible," which recreates a critical framework for setting up an architectural theory of atmosphere of an experiential identity, inspired by notions of a (neuro)biological origin — derived from a previously metabolised transition of the phenomenological and aesthetics repertoire. Specifically, four scientific principles are examined: the multisensory nature of spatial perceptual processes; the dynamics of embodiment, which highlights the crucial role of the body-brain-mind unit entrenched in its environment of movement and interaction; the emotional content of the architectural experience; and the phenomenon of emotional and physiological empathy.

I
A Definition Lacking Definition

1. *Rooms and Atmospheres*

When we enter a room, we become aware of the atmosphere.

The room is a very small part of the architectural score. It is an elementary, but complete form of architecture (Ottolini 2010), a unit of space and air, which accommodates and assists the complex rituals of living. Enclosed within precise margins that are solid, continuous, or fragmented (or rather: a series of walls, floor, ceiling, windows, and doors); it originates empty, to then be equipped and personalised by its occupants, who according to their experiences and necessities, fill it with furniture, objects, and domestic goods. The dimensions, shape, and decoration vary depending on period, cultural inclination, and socio-economic situation. Differences in taste and elective affinities are particularly recognisable in the bedroom — the living cell where we sleep, or simply spend time. "Many roads," explains the French historian Michelle Perrot, "lead to the bedroom: sleep, rest, birth, death, desire, love, meditation, reading, writing, search of self, God, reclusion (whether desired or endured), illness" (2018, 1). The bedroom represents the most remote and separate island in our personal geography, which for hours every day, we warm with our bodies and our emotions. "The bedroom protects us, our thoughts, our letters, our furniture, our belongings. Like a rampart, it repels the invader. It welcomes us, like a refuge" (Perrot, 3). More than any other, it is the place in which the spatial dynamics tend to express their human dimension.

In an attempt to identify the constituent elements of a room, the primordial and essential nucleus of architecture, first to emerge would be those that we define the *fundamental elements of architecture*, namely the physical components that have kept an identifiable and significant consistency of use in the history of the discipline (Scelsi 2021).[1] Examples are doors, windows, walls, ceilings, ramps, corridors, and fireplaces (Koolhaas et al. 2014) or again, balconies, staircases, and vaults (Ponti 1960). They design and materialise the confines of the space. These confines are endowed with thickness, consistency, weight, and materiality; confines that are concrete, visible, tangible, and quantifiable.

But there is a "but." Or better, also there is an "also." In the sense that if there are a perimeter, sides, and a shell, there must *also* be a content: an emptiness that becomes substance. "The emptiness, the void, is what does the vessel's holding," as exemplified by Martin Heidegger (1975, 169) in the famous metaphor of the jug, with which he calls into question the being of the object.

Slowly moving on, and using a vocabulary that is more consistent with and familiar to those who inhabit the architectural arena, we can evoke a phrase by the Japanese writer Okakura Kakuzō, which struck Frank Lloyd Wright when he read his *The Book of Tea* (1906): "the reality of a room," notes Wright, "[is] to be found in the space enclosed by the roof and walls, not in the roof and walls themselves" (Kaufmann and Raeburn 1960, 300). Bruno Zevi explains why.

> Architecture [...] does not consist in the sum of the width, length and height of the structural elements that enclose space, but in the void itself, the enclosed space in which the human lives and moves. [...] To grasp space, to know how to *see* it, is the key to the understanding of building. (Zevi [1948] 1993, 22–23: original italics)

The architect must learn to engage in architectural emptiness, the source of spatial experience, since it deals with a phenomenon that, concentrated solely in architecture, constitutes "its specific character" (Zevi, 27). Le

---

[1] The German architect and architectural theoretician Gottfried Semper identified *four* primigenial elements of architecture. "The first sign of settlement and rest after the hunt, the battle, and wandering in the desert is today, as when the first men lost paradise, the setting up of the fireplace and the lighting of the reviving, warming, and food-preparing flame. [...] [The *hearth*] is the first and most important, the *moral* element of architecture. Around it were grouped the three other elements: the *roof*, the *enclosure*, and the *mound*, the protecting negations or defenders of the hearth's flame against the three hostile elements of nature" ([1851] 1989 as reprinted in 2018, 22: original italics).

Corbusier spoke on this topic at his third conference with the Faculty of Exact Sciences in Buenos Aires, more than ninety years ago.[2]

> Architecture is an act of conscious willpower.
> To create architecture *is to put in order*.
> Put what in order? Functions and objects. To occupy space with buildings and with roads. To create containers to shelter people and useful transportation to get to them. To act on our minds by the cleverness of the solutions, on our senses by the forms proposed and by the distances we are obliged to walk. To move by the play of perceptions to which we are sensitive, and which we cannot avoid. Spaces, dimensions and forms, interior spaces and interior forms, interior pathways and exterior forms, and exterior spaces — quantities, weights, distances, atmospheres, it is with these that we act. (Le Corbusier 2015, 68–70: original italics)

In a nutshell, Le Corbusier's lecture on the essence of daily architectural practice could be condensed into a highly evocative image: "Architecture is […] atmospheres."[3] As much the material components that configure and functionalize the space (namely objects, buildings, roads) as the emotional tension the space emanates (atmospheres) are necessary to define the identity of the staged architectural event. They are complementary tools that assimilate and reinforce each other. In order for the atmospheric vocation of architecture to manifest itself, the presence of the subject who experiences it must be guaranteed. We need an agent who enters into direct contact with the domain of suggestions and spatial stimuli that are radiated by the context. Which is to say, there must be the required "right angle," to use another expression dear to Le Corbusier (1955): the geometric result of the meeting of vertical and horizontal lines that symbolize respectively the active man taking possession of the space and the irregular and cracked surface of the ground on which he moves. Only in this way does architecture come alive and become *atmosphere* — lived space, living space. Only like this can a room be conceived as a unit of atmospheric space. It is a question of beginning to read the architectural score of a perspective that other

---

2   In the autumn of 1929, during his long travels on the continent of South America, Le Corbusier was the key player in a cycle of ten conferences in Argentina, organised by three institutions: the Friends of the Arts, the Faculty of Exact Sciences, and the Friends of the City. The third encounter, from which the passage comes, was entitled *Architecture in Everything, City Planning in Everything*. Numerous architecture students attended the lesson.

3   To explain the emotional content of architecture, even Thomas Thiis-Evensen, Christian Norberg-Schulz's pupil, underlined that "Le Corbusier saw moods as the essence of architecture" (1987, 15).

disciplines (first of all the aesthetic-philosophical fields) have perfected from the second half of the twentieth century (Griffero and Moretti 2018) and that places affective excess of corporeal-spatial perception at the centre of discussion (De Matteis 2021).

2. Blurred Certainties

Every epoch has its references and elects its masters. For Ludwig Mies van der Rohe, "Building Art is the spatially apprehended will of the epoch. Alive. Changing. New" ([1923] 1991, 241).

Initially as students, later as architects, my generation grew up in the cult of the poetics of the Swiss architect Peter Zumthor. His figure established itself in the mid-nineties with the design of the Thermal Baths at Vals,[4] a peaceful holiday location nestled in the Alpine landscape of the Grisons: an authentic "monument of European architectural history," as the project was hailed in *Domus*, a year after its inauguration (Steiner 1997, 27). The principle merit that should be recognised at the thermal baths in Vals is that "they were the first material contribution to the recent debate on an architecture that primarily appealed to the senses" (Wegerhoff 2016, 119). Peter Zumthor dominated the international scene in the early years of the third millennium, anointed in 2009 when he was awarded the prestigious — or, at least mediatically resonant — Pritzker Architecture Prize. The works he designed[5] became icons of a new aesthetic, playing on sensory equilibrium and the integration between the individual and their architectonic surroundings. "It is hard to speak about the work of Peter Zumthor with due detachment," admits the architectural critic Friedrich Achleitner. "His buildings call for an unconditional willingness to get involved" (1997, 52). To cite an exemplary case of his design philosophy, in 2007 Zumthor completed the field chapel dedicated to Bruder Klaus[6] in Mechernich, Germany, commissioned by Hermann-Josef and Trude Scheidtweiler, an elderly farming couple who wanted to thank God for the long life He have given them.[7]

4　See Zumthor and Mostafavi (1996); Zumthor (1997); Zumthor and Hauser (2007).
5　See Zumthor (1998); Durisch (2014).
6　Nicholas of Flüe (also known as Brother Klaus) was a Swiss hermit, today worshipped by the Catholic Church as a saint, and the patron of Switzerland.
7　See Baglione (2007); Casciani (2007).

A Definition Lacking Definition

The small chapel stands, silent, in the middle of the verdant fields of the Eifel, looking somewhat like a monolithic shell, welded to the ground. However, unlike a normal shell, smooth and shiny on the inside, the building has a polished amber-coloured exterior mantle that encloses a ridged, rough, and seasoned cavity. A prism on a pentagonal plan, with irregular sides, shrouds a sinuous cavern, whose curvilinear walls have been cropped on a temporary formwork of a hundred and twelve tree trunks, placed in a cone. The space between the two shells has been saturated with coats of dripped concrete, twenty-four to be exact, poured in layers of about fifty centimetres, each marking a day's work. After the requisite drying time for the concrete mass, the internal formwork was set on fire and left to burn for three weeks: a coarse skin of a rich brown colour surfaced, scratched with the marks of the fire and smelling of ashes.

The dimensions of the building are intimate, and considerately contained: twelve metres high, with sides that vary between about three and eight metres long. The architect chose to use natural and indigenous materials: the tree trunks come from a nearby forest belonging to the clients, and gravel from a local river was used in the cement mix. The light, besides leaking delicately into the interior, alights on a constellation of three hundred crystal beads, placed to cover the stay rods left open in the concrete walls, and falls copiously through the mystical central oculus that opens up to the sky: a slight breeze, gentle rain, rays of sunshine, and the glow of stars are free to drop to the lead floor. As Tadao Ando suggests, questioning the function of architecture as a vehicle for interaction with the natural environment, "abstracted nature — such as air, water, earth and light — and natural phenomena — such as rain, snow, sky, sea, forest and mountains — empower architecture to materialise the intangible" (2021, 1). This is precisely what happens in the work of Peter Zumthor. Here, concrete, glass, and fire (Baglione 2006), coming together in a harmony of materials, provide an extraordinary response — solid, tangible, and architectonic — to the question from which we trace the beginnings of atmospheric research in architecture. Zumthor himself brings this question to the discussion table: *what do we mean when we speak of architectural quality?*

> It is a question I have little difficulty in answering. Quality in architecture does not — not to me anyway — mean inclusion in architectural guides or histories of architecture or getting my work into this or that publication. Quality architecture to me is when a building manages to move me. [...] One word for it is atmosphere. (Zumthor 2006, 11)

Atmosphere, which Peter Zumthor (nearly eighty years after Le Corbusier)[8] raises to a founding act in architectural practice, is, quintessentially, an intangible condition of the architectural space; and, being intangible, seems evasive and hard to translate and communicate, because it involves sensations that — in determining architectural quality — transcend the visual dimension. The Western cultural code, dominated by the supremacy of sight over the other senses (Levin 1993), bases the practice and fruition of architecture on an obsessively oculocentric approach (Pallasmaa 2012a). Le Corbusier's message is clear (1931, 29): "architecture is the masterly, correct and magnificent play of masses brought together in light. Our eyes are made to see forms in light." However, the atmospheric aura shies away from the sovereignty of the eye: we lap at it by means of different sensory and perceptual channels; atmosphere pervades the spatial organism from which it is irradiated, and touches the individual in a synaesthetic and integrated manner. Thus causing the "play of masses" to lose clarity and transform into "ineffable space": "then a boundless depth opens up, effaces the walls, drives away contingent presences, *accomplishes the miracle of ineffable space* [...] the consummation of plastic emotion" (Le Corbusier 1948, 8: original italics). One leaves the confines of Euclidean geometry and finds oneself immersed in the atmospheric dimension. In "a state that is hardly defined, not because it is rare and unusual but, on the contrary, because it is as omnipresent — even though at times unnoticed — as the emotive situation" (Griffero 2014a, 1). "The atmospheres, so obvious as to be imperceptible, in which we live, move, and have our being," (Sloterdijk 2016, 62) prompt our daily life. Atmospheric contact is a sensation that everyone knows and to which everyone refers, more or less directly and consciously.

We speak of the tense atmosphere of a meeting, the light-hearted atmosphere of a day, the gloomy atmosphere of a vault; we refer to the atmosphere of a

---

8   Le Corbusier and Zumthor share Swiss origins: the former was born in 1887 at La Chaux-de-Fonds, in the francophone region of the Jura; the latter was born in 1943 in Basel, homonymous capital of the canton, of German cultural mould. Although their expressive repertoires have rarely been compared, they share profound similarities of approach to the emotive-atmospheric qualities of constructed space. Interviewed in 2004 for *Casabella*, Peter Zumthor refers to the concept of *ineffable space* put forward by Le Corbusier (Stec 2004, 91) as "a beautiful idea." The concept is based on the conviction that objects, when they resonate with each other, irradiate a special harmony, introducing a fourth dimension, not included in those of Descartes, which becomes the domain of aesthetic emotions (Le Corbusier 1948).

city, a restaurant, a landscape. [...] An extraordinarily rich vocabulary may be used to describe it: cheerful, sublime, melancholy, stuffy, oppressive, tense, uplifting. We also speak of the atmosphere of the 1920s, of a pretty bourgeois atmosphere, of the atmosphere of power. (Böhme 1998, 112)

We could even go so far as to say that human beings *breathe* the atmospheric charge of the environments they inhabit. "They are rooted in" the atmospheres of those places, states Frank Lloyd Wright, "just as a plant is in the soil in which it is planted" (1954, 135). Despite this link being so intense and customary, as though it were a spontaneous and necessary form of *symbiosis*, explaining it is not obvious: when we speak of atmospheres, meaning and sign overlap in a hazy horizon of interpretation. "The question 'what is an atmosphere?'," asserts Tonino Griffero, "is still — perhaps necessarily, given the reifying presupposition of the question? — not answered satisfactorily" (2014a, 1–2).

3. *A Challenge to the Vague*

The immediate intelligibility of a word seems to vanish when we try to give it an exact and unequivocal definition. Such a mechanism is fully confirmed with the atmospheric construction. Mark Wigley forcefully reaffirms this in an article from 1998, which over the years has become a milestone in atmospheric research in the field of architectonics.

Atmospheric effects cannot be avoided. They permeate architecture. Architecture is defined by atmosphere. [...] At the same time, those who embrace effect cannot approach atmosphere directly — cannot point to it, cannot teach it. Atmosphere escapes the discourse about it. By definition, it lacks definition. It is precisely that which escapes analysis. Any specific proposal for constructing atmosphere, no matter how changeable or indeterminate, is no longer atmospheric. [...] Atmosphere may be the core of architecture but it is a core that cannot simply be addressed or controlled. (Wigley 1998a, 27)

In the first instance, what makes the analysis of atmosphere complex is its vagueness. Vagueness that manifests itself on three different levels: semantic, ontological, and epistemic (Rauh 2017). By *semantic vagueness* we mean "the indistinctness, in principle or in fact, of terms or concepts" (Rauh, §13); *ontological vagueness* alludes to a "vagueness as an element of the world and of reality" (§14); while *epistemic vagueness* refers to "a deficiency of knowledge, in principle or in fact, regarding the object under discussion" (§15). This book aims to clarify the atmospheric phenomenon in architecture setting out from this basis: the impalpability of its substance. An initial step is to address the presumed diffidence with regard to the possibility of a stipulated definition and to go beyond the sense of disorientation produced by the vast existing domain of the notion of atmosphere, whose great range is attributable precisely to the lack of a precise semantic delimitation.[9]

There are many themes in architecture that — even basing oneself on shared references — prove to be intrinsically elusive and weakly formizable; for example, consider the *empty space*.

> Emptiness and constructed material form the polarities at the basis of architecture. [...] Like water or smoke passing through the fingers, emptiness seems to be fatally destined to escape definition. This is why the job of building emptiness — the void that worries or moves us, that calms or saddens us, that encourages us to an action or to frame a subject, with which we impose order or purify ourselves — holds undeniable interest. (Espuelas 1999, 9)

There are numerous possible strategies to chip away at the barrier of ineffability, or to be more exact, there are numerous levels of study to which one might take the search for a definition. Focusing on the abovementioned experience of emptiness, two main methodological solutions of opposing analytical intensity present themselves. On the one hand, an elaboration of extended and all-encompassing readings aimed at "unveiling the void, or rather, the voids in architecture that bring their own qualities in different nuances (expressive, regulatory, psychological, symbolic, etc.) to define space" (Espuelas, 10). On the other hand, more evanescent and tautological readings prevail, in which the discussion evaporates in the claim that, to carry out its function, emptiness should not be filled, but accepted as it is; there follows, in the latter case, the declaration of axioms, that — however suggestive — impart apparent truths rather than explanations. "Where there is nothing, everything is possible. Where there is architecture, nothing (else) is possible": for example, is the provocative warning of Rem Koolhaas (1985, 199).

In any case, we need to admit the innate condition of indeterminacy that distinguishes the argument in hand and choose how to proceed: whether to attempt to codify it, conferring a systemic character on it; or to leave it open

---

9   See chapters II "Roots" and III "Atlas of Atmospheres."

and never completely graspable in its subtleties. The challenge undertaken here has been to exaggerate the former position, not only identifying a definition of the concept of architectural atmosphere, but also taking the risk of ascribing to it a sense system obedient to scientific criteria. In other words, I asked myself if it were possible to formalize such an intrinsically vague concept, until now outlined by the architectural discipline above all through metaphor and "ineffable" expressions, synthesizing a scientifically objective formula, or a model that is employable as a general rule. As a result, I rejected the authoritative advice of Professor Mark Wigley. Among the first experts to interest themselves in the theme of atmosphere in the architectural field, at the end of the nineties (1998a), Wigley maintains that we cannot directly approach the essence of atmosphere, nor can we determine its identity, much less reveal it to others. As will be shown below, "atmosphere" is a decidedly broad term, which is spacious and employed increasingly. There is the sense that it must involve rigorous study capable of taking root as a tight and original reference, within the ecosystem of research and publications on the theme of atmosphere that, particularly in these years, is seeing a significant development.[10]

From a functional point of view, to relieve the stranglehold of the ineffability of the atmospheric nature, I have tried to establish a hierarchy among the different orders of vagueness. In the first place, I have considered the question put forward by philosopher Tonino Griffero in the introduction to his treatise originally entitled *Atmosferologia* (atmospherology, in English), regarding scientific research into atmosphere.

> One might wonder [...] whether [the atmospheres] constitute a semantic or *de dicto* vagueness (the atmospheric description designates a given situation in a vague way) or instead [...] a metaphysical or *de re* vagueness (the atmospheric description designates a vague entity in a precise way), analogous to that attributable to many other quasi-things, such as colours, shadows, etc. (Griffero 2014a, 7)

The choice, moreover the one recommended by Griffero, fell upon the second position: establishing that *the atmospheric description designates a vague entity in a precise way*. Hence, in the light of a purposely coined definition — which at least aims to overcome the level of semantic vagueness[11] — the personal diagnosis of architectural atmospheres

---

10 See chapter IV "Atmospheric Revival."
11 See chapter V "To Perceive the Invisible."

conceives the atmospheric medium as a vehicle to articulate the indefinite and formless content that feeds the phenomenal-perceptual reaction of the individual in the act of immersing in their architectonic surroundings. In essence, the decision is to relegate prevalent impulses of vagueness to the ontological plain. This strategy follows a fundamental teaching of Gernot Böhme, who for years used the concept of atmosphere as the key to a special interpretation of the aesthetic experience.

> Atmospheres are indeterminate above all as regards their ontological status. We are not sure whether we should attribute them to the objects or environments from which they proceed or to the subjects who experience them. We are also unsure where they are. They seem to fill the space with a certain tone of feeling like a haze. (Böhme 1993, 114)

Meanwhile, the path of research undertaken imposes a less confused and incoherent cognitive layout, that disentangles — as far as possible — the climate of epistemic vagueness in which designers and researchers of the architectural discipline currently move.

4. Atmospheric Code

Having established the intrinsic premise of ineffability of the atmospheric code, one can move onto an examination of the substantial set of factors that render its description and interpretation complex.

First unknown: invisibility

In the first place, it must be stressed that atmosphere is invisible. Located as it is, at the limits of perception, woken by heterogeneous sensory stimuli so closely interconnected that they are hard to separate and identify. From the time of classical Greece, the eye asserts a hegemonic role in the processes of mediation and comprehension of physical reality, as it is reputed to be the privileged organ in the construction of consciousness. "This is how it is: he who sees has acquired knowledge, we say, of that which he has seen; for it is agreed that sight and perception and knowledge are all the same [...] 'does not see' is the same as 'does not know,' if it is true that seeing is knowing" — so Plato ([fourth century BC] 1921, 84–85:

164 a–b),[12] in the words of an aging Socrates, condensed the sensualist thought of the Sophists. The Western world has inherited this propensity for empirical rationality: escaping visual recognition, it is as if atmosphere also evades rational comprehension. A geometric-linear reading of space, based on mere visual significance is no longer sufficient if the intention is to analyse the atmospheric dimension and its emotional reverberations.

Certain authors have dealt with the apparently paradoxical question of rendering visible the invisible body of architectural atmosphere, seeking simplified models in its multifactorial structure. Among them Malte Wagenfeld, researcher at the Royal Melbourne Institute of Technology (RMIT), who for several years curated the project entitled *Aesthetics of Air* (2013), an interesting experimental investigation into atmospheric phenomena, focused on their aeriform essence. Atmosphere is understood as a combination of sensory perceptions stimulated by the air; which is to say: by its movements, temperature, level of humidity, the sounds and smells it carries, its density, weight, and so on. Since air is, by its very constitution, invisible, Wagenfeld uses different techniques and approaches (such as laser visualization systems) "to 'reveal' air as a visible presence in a space — as an observable material" (2015a, 9). In principle, to sound the aerial domain, hypothesized as a "dynamic amalgam" of interacting forces and energies "rather than as a material thing" (Wagenfeld, 10), he concentrated on direct observation of movements of the air out in the open. He chose natural spaces, such as the Melbourne Botanical Gardens, which allowed him access to surfaces and objects that were sensible to the passage of air (mainly: blades of grass, leafy branches, and expanses of water); then, he moved on to making films, reproducing — in slow motion — minimal oscillations and variations in movement; finally, he mapped the topography of swirling air currents in a closed environment, making use of laser and fogger.[13] However reductive and imperfect, these initial attempts to depict air physically, provide a valid point of departure in the research for methods and instruments that permit the assembly of empirical applications for the study of atmosphere in architectonic spaces.

---

12 Plato. 1921. *Theaetetus — Sophist*. Trans. by H.N. Fowler. The Loeb Classical Library, 123. London: William Heinemann — New York, NY: G.P. Putnam's Sons. The date of the *Theaetetus* is uncertain, but it cannot be one of the early dialogues. The mention of the Athenian army at Corinth makes any date much earlier than 390 BC impossible (see "Introduction to the Theaetetus," 5).
13 Nebulizers that produce clouds of vapour thick enough to resemble fog.

Second unknown: incorporeality

Atmosphere is incorporeal, which is different from being invisible, and still more indefinable on a level of perception.[14] Atmosphere cannot be touched, isolated, or attributed to a specific concrete source. It is abstract. Unlike other sensory experiences, it acts above all without the subject being aware and leaves no trace for autonomous considerations with regard to timeline, cause/effect, or analogy/similarity, which intervene between the suggestions caught. An example helps clarify this last reflection: imagine hearing a door slam in the other room.

> In this case here, the sound is instantly recognized as the sound of the door, and is immediately associated with the material built element that causes the sonic sensation, and which ultimately *is* the sound. [...] The sound of the door (although it is a non-material fluid element of space like the atmosphere) is instantly recognized and identified with the door; there is not very much beyond this specific understanding of the sound. On the contrary, though, the atmosphere of a place (the sensation of a particular atmosphere) cannot be easily identified with one, specific element of a space; it is a result of several parameters and conditions. (Karandinou 2013, 21: original italics)

Atmosphere's condition of immateriality makes it (at first sight) impossible to identify, measure, and chart. What technologies, from among those traditionally available, can be employed to analyse it? It is unthinkable to consider the use of tools typical in meteorological practice, such as thermometers, anemometers, or barometers: efficient for gathering numerical data to monitor the chemical, electric, and thermodynamic processes of atmospheric flow, but incapable of interpreting perceptual qualities. Logically, the classical techniques of architectural representation, such as graphical transpositions of plans, sections, and perspective views, can also be excluded. New experimental methods are required. At the beginning of the sixties, Louis Kahn reflects on the immaterial as follows:

> This is a question of the unmeasurable and the measurable. Nature, physical nature, is measurable. Feeling and dream has no measure, has no language, and everyone's dream is singular. Everything that is made however obeys the laws of nature. [...] "Then," said the young architect, "what should be the discipline, what should be the ritual that brings one closer to the psyche? For in this aura

---

14 Air, for example, is also invisible, but it has its own sensorially perceptible consistency, indicated by the pressure it exercises on the skin, by alternating temperatures, and by smells with which it is impregnated.

of no material and no language, I feel *man* truly is." (Kahn 1960, radio lecture, as reprinted in 1962, 114: italics not original)

Innovative paradigms to understand the *unmeasurably human* are today offered by a synergy of disciplines,[15] which explore the human dimension of the vast panorama of spatial experiences. Such disciplinary hints seem to be able to produce an answer, that is also operative, to the affirmation of the physical incongruity in which atmosphere gains corporeality, and therefore weight, from the moment that material loses its tangible concreteness, letting itself be permeated by the affective surplus of the stimuli perceived by the subject.

Third unknown: uncontrollability

Atmosphere has no physical confines: it cannot be precisely located or circumscribed in the space enclosed between the walls of a room. "Like clouds in the sky," atmospheres "are ever forming and reforming, appearing and disappearing, never finished or at rest" (Asu Schroer and Schmitt 2018, 1). They constitute the perspective of sensory-emotional interaction of the individual with a specific spatiality, composed as much by the architectonic elements that make it up as by the emptiness modelled by them. Although uncontrollable, atmosphere has real effects that we try to gather, define, and set a perimeter around. In other words, we are attempting to find an answer to the question that the academic Dora Zhang asks, in the course of her inquiry into the social and political importance that atmospheric phenomena assume in daily life: "what difference does an atmosphere make to an environment, a situation, or a horizon of possible action?" and "where exactly does it reside?" (2018, 121).

It is in the voids that mark out a place that atmosphere acquires its form, never stable, never definitively delimited — in constant equilibrium between the sensibility of the experiencing subject and the solicitations exercised by the architectonically organized environment. As Tonino Griffero observes, taking up a passage from the German philosopher Michael Hauskeller, it is conceivable that atmosphere also has confines, beyond which its influence ceases. "A manner of thinking probably suggested by the model of smell" (Griffero 2012, 188): indeed, like smell, "the atmosphere of a

---

15 E.g., experimental phenomenology, environmental psychology, and cognitive science, among others.

thing extends as far as its presence makes a difference" (Hauskeller 1995, 33).[16] The concept of difference, or of perceptual gap, is also put forward by the German sociologist and philosopher Niklas Luhmann: "atmosphere is a kind of excess effect caused by the difference between places" (2000, 112). This *difference* has an effect on the sensory-perceptive spectrum of the spatially immersed individual, given that, as Juhani Pallasmaa explains in his accessible breviary of architectural phenomenology, "the boundary line between the self and the world is identified by our senses" (Pallasmaa and Zambelli 2020, 123).

Fourth unknown: complexity

Atmosphere is complex, or rather it grafts onto an articulated palimpsest of variables, in continual evolution, held in a relationship of reciprocal tension in their proteiform heterogeneity. It is not a question of mere physical-environmental variables, such as temperature, humidity, or level of oxygen, which can be controlled with great precision. No, qualitative variables are operating, of subjective origin and intricate valuation. Above all, in immediate spatial contact, a synergy of sensory perceptions intervenes, fused among them.

> The judgement of environmental character is a complex multi-sensory fusion of countless factors which are immediately and synthetically grasped as an overall atmosphere, ambience, feeling or mood. [...] An atmospheric perception also involves judgements beyond the five Aristotelian senses, such as sensations of orientation, gravity, balance, stability, motion, duration, continuity, scale and illumination. (Pallasmaa 2014a, 230–231)

The matter is further complicated if the enquiry is moved onto a higher interpretive level, which is to say poetic and figurative; in the major part of cases, when we talk of atmosphere in architecture we do so in a metaphorical key, tapping into an imagination of greatly expanded references. "The concept of atmosphere is interesting," notes Professor Ben Anderson, a cultural-political geographer, "because it holds a series of opposites — presence and absence, materiality and ideality, definite and indefinite, singularity and generality — in a relation of tension" (2009, 77). The list of dichotomies could go on, increasing the level of vagueness that characterizes the atmospheric construct: internal and external, private and public, ordinary and extraordinary, and so on. It is precisely this ambiguity

---

16 As cited and translated in Griffero 2014a, 126 n. 81.

that makes the notion of atmosphere interesting from an anthropological point of view, for it allows us "to see the atmosphere simultaneously as an object of perception, as the result of interaction, as well as an artefact" (Gruppuso 2018, 47).

At the point in which we recognise the process of atmospheric suggestion as something produced by the human being, design factors can finally step in. Indeed, it is the architectonic landscape, with its voids and fulls, that stages the atmospheric artifice — coordinating different sources of emotional impression — that combine together to set up a unitary spatial effect. The design variables, states Le Corbusier,[17] are numerous.

> To the young student, I should ask: how do you make a door? What size? Where do you put it? How do you make a window? But, in fact, what is a window for? Do you really know why windows are made? If you know, tell us. [...] At what point of a bedroom do you open a door? Why there and not elsewhere? Ah, you seem to have many solutions? You are right, there are many possible solutions and each gives a different architectural sensation. Ah, you realize that different solutions are the very basis of architecture? Depending on the way you enter a room, depending on the place of the door in the wall, you feel a certain sensation and the wall that you have perceived also takes a very different character. You feel that there is architecture. [...] Another equally serious question: where do you open your window? You notice, that depending on where light comes from, you feel such or such a sensation? Well, then draw all the different ways possible to open a window and you will tell me which are better. [...] Oh, you can buy a thick notebook for this work, you shall need a lot of pages. (Le Corbusier 2015, 222)

The *atmospheric continuum*, needing to mediate this multifactorial nature, is necessarily assimilated as an area of approximation. It stands as a sort of *in-between* dimension, absorbing incessant variations and contaminations, and softening spatial sharp points in gradual, subtler passages. "Atmosphere would not benefit from an excessive formal vividness," states Tonino Griffero (2014a, 6 n. 20), to the extent that atmospheres might be understood as "the more positively active the more they are evanescent" (Griffero, 6). Some architects choose — in a pragmatic manner — to adopt the *in-between model* as a system to compensate the

---

17 The following passage is an extract from the lecture *The World City and Some Perhaps Untimely Considerations* (originally entitled *Si je devais enseigner l'architecture?*), which Le Corbusier presented at the Faculty of Exact Sciences of Buenos Aires on Thursday 17 October 1929.

antithetical elements in the space, as a working instrument to synthesize the multiple and the complex, like a sieve to sift the emotional particles triggered. Gradation becomes a recurrent design strategy, for example, in the poetics of the Japanese architect Sou Fujimoto, who designs installations, such as the 2013 pavilion for London's Serpentine Gallery,[18] in which "the whole atmosphere made by grids [is] blurring and ambiguous, like trees or a forest or clouds."[19]

> Gradation will become the keyword for the future of architecture. For instance, there are infinite colorific degrees between white and black, and innumerable values between 1 and 0. Conventional architecture systematizes our world in the name of "functionalism," as if clearly differentiated into black and white. [...] Unlike the Internet, space is not capable of switching from 0 to 1 instantaneously. Conversely, the allure of space must lay in its ability to actualize in reality the possibilities of a gradation between 0 and 1. (Fujimoto 2010, 199)

The score of tonalities becomes the filter of preference to read complexity that inhabits the disassembled and rarefied territory of the atmospheric event. It suggests that we observe the architectonic scene with a "limitless" eye, trying to read it not in single details, but gathering the mixture of colours, textures, and gradations of light.

Fifth unknown: mutability

Atmosphere is mutable: it is continually changing, innervated as it is, with regular instability. It is the fruit of the subject-stimulus situational influence, or rather of a function of interdependency that involves the

---

18 Every year, the Serpentine Gallery, famous contemporary art gallery in London's Kensington Gardens, Hyde Park, sets up a temporary pavilion on the lawn by the gallery entrance, to house the rich palimpsest of summer cultural events from July to October. Each time the design of the Serpentine Gallery Pavilion is assigned to a different architect, distinguished in the international arena but who has never built anything on English soil. The prestigious cycle was inaugurated by Zaha Hadid in 2000. Peter Zumthor was responsible for the pavilion in 2011 alongside the Dutch landscape designer Piet Oudolf; see 2011. "Peter Zumthor: Serpentine Gallery Pavilion 2011." *A+u. Architecture and Urbanism* 492 (Art and Architecture): 16–23.

19 Sou Fujimoto describes his project for the Serpentine Pavilion in an interview for the magazine *Dezeen*. See Etherington, Rose. 2013. "Serpentine Gallery Pavilion 2013 by Sou Fujimoto." *Dezeen* (online), 4 June 2013: n.p. — www.dezeen.com, last accessed 20 April 2021.

A Definition Lacking Definition 31

spatial as much as the temporal dimension: a genuine *hic et nunc*, in the literal sense. As the architectural historian Alberto Pérez-Gómez emphasises, "atmospheres are spatial phenomena, but always intertwined with temporality; they are never 'outside' time" (2016, 18). They mirror the identity of a specific fragment of time, whether is it attributable to a meteorological source[20] or assigned to the personal sphere of the individual, of which it scans every activity, physical and mental.[21] In this last case, a factor that has a strong impact on atmospheric impressionability is the link with memory. The time of inhabited space is the time that measures human actions; and does it in a non-linear and discontinued manner that is incessantly swayed by the influence of memory. The influence of every private past, and the memories carried within it, is powerful and inevitable: assailing and conditioning the individual sensibility, leaving no margin of defence or control, at least initially. For Peter Zumthor, the virginity of atmospheric contact fades with the appearance of memory, which arms reflection with involuntarily preconceived personal convictions. For this reason, the atmosphere of a place undergoes sudden changes, according to mnemic input, that can be inherent as much in the overall architectural disposition as in any detail of it, however small.

> When I think about architecture, images come into my mind. Many of these images are connected with my training and work as an architect. They contain the professional knowledge about architecture that I have gathered over the years. Some of the other images have to do with my childhood. There was a time when I experienced architecture without thinking about it. [...] Memories like these contain the deepest architectural experience that I know. They are the reservoirs of the architectural atmospheres and images that I explore in my work as an architect. (Zumthor 1988, 9–10)

The assault of memory — guardian of lived experiences — is instinctive and instantaneous. Thus, even on a temporal level, atmospheres show labile boundaries, which can dissolve or thicken in an instant, with no warning, like gassy swarms. Once again it is Peter Zumthor who explains it well.

> I enter a building, see a room, and — in the fraction of a second — have this feeling about it. We perceive atmosphere through our emotional sensibility — a form of perception that works incredibly quickly, and which we humans evidently need to help us survive. [...] Something inside us tells us an enormous amount

---

20 Time, that is, defined by climatic geography, seasonal intermittence, or by circadian rhythm.
21 Namely: absolute time, relative time; cultural time, interior time.

straight away. We are capable of immediate appreciation, of a spontaneous emotional response, of rejecting things in a flash. (Zumthor 2006, 13)

To sum up: mutability and instantaneity mark the atmospheric equilibrium, resulting from the balance of power between the components deployed within the individual domain and spatial contingencies, which charge the surroundings with an explosive reactive potential. The intervention of memory unleashes retrospective and future projections that shake up our sensibility, de-stabilising it until it reaches a new emotional equilibrium, different from the initial condition.

Sixth unknown: subjectivity

Atmosphere is, by its status, subjective: it arises with the individual experiencing it, but it is not traceable only to their state of mind. "Atmosphere is the prototypical 'between'-phenomenon. [...] [It] is something between the subject and the object" (1998, 112). This interpretative approach comes from the aesthetics theories formulated, from the last decade of the twentieth century, by the German philosopher Gernot Böhme,[22] who has provided many of the ideas on which the preparatory analysis of this book is based.

> Atmosphere is the shared reality of the perceiver and the perceived. It is the reality of the perceived as the sphere of its presence and the reality of the perceiver insofar as he or she, in sensing the atmosphere, is bodily present in a particular way. (Böhme 2017b, 23–24)

It is impossible to think of an atmospheric event separated from the individual immersed in the architectonic context or detached from their mental state, from the interior processes that animate their sensibility (as much sensory as affective), and from the episodes of life that develop their personal past. A symbiotic balance surfaces that rests "at the threshold between biography and world of facts, things and situations" (Hasse 1994,

---

[22] On the theme of atmosphere, Gernot Böhme has produced a robust anthology of monographic works: see Böhme 1995a, 2001, 2006, 2017a; besides numerous papers, among which the following texts are of particular interest for the architectural discipline: Böhme 1991, 1993, 1995b, 1998, 2005, 2013a, 2013b, 2013c, 2013d, 2014. Two recent publications translated and collected some of his writings, for the first time making them accessible to an English-reading public: Böhme 2017b, 2017c.

58).[23] Atmospheres are nothing in the absence of a sentient subject and are perceived only in subjective experience. Although unable to exist independently of the subject, they can however prescind from the subject's awareness. The famous experiment by the American philosopher Thomas Nagel, in which we are invited to imagine what it would feel like to be a bat, can help us better understand how delicate it is to investigate the intrinsically subjective nature of atmospheric experience.

> Every subjective phenomenon is essentially connected with a single point of view [...]. Our own experience provides the basic material for our imagination, whose range is therefore limited [...]. I want to know what it is like for a *bat* to be a bat. Yet if I try to imagine this, I am restricted to the resources of my own mind, and those resources are inadequate to the task. I cannot perform it either by imaging additions to my present experience, or by imagining segments gradually subtracted from it, or by imagining some combination of additions, subtractions, and modifications. [...] The best evidence would come from the experiences of bats, if we only knew what they were like. So if extrapolation from our own case is involved in the idea of what it is like to be a bat, the extrapolation must be incompletable (Nagel 1974, 437; 439: original italics)

To understand what an individual feels, on a subjective level, is not a simple question to answer. At most, one might try to imagine, but we would anyhow only obtain a partial, approximate, and perhaps hasty description. Such an attempt would be more efficient if the observer could have a similar conscious experience: "it is often possible to take up a point of view other than one's own," concedes Nagel. However, "the more different from oneself the other experiencer is, the less success one can expect with this enterprise" (1974, 441–442). The atmospheric dynamics, with its promiscuous swirl between subjective and objective poles, or rather between a subjective character of the experience and an impulse of a factual nature, matches mental processes to physical processes and confronts specifically human points of view with material-spatial mechanisms.

Seventh unknown: immaturity

Atmosphere is immature, crude, awaiting a suitable education. In other words, it has not yet been refined (in adequate measure) in study models or formalised in operating codes, much less through the classical analytical methods — verbal or graphical — on which the practice of

---

23 As cited and translated in Griffero 2014a, 121.

architecture is based. As for other concepts that belong to the discipline, which are structurally vague but amply shared (for example, the analogy), it may be noted that "the gulf is immense between theory and practice" (Melandri 1968, 11). Until a few years ago, the disciplines of architectural design have not shown themselves particularly interested in organizing atmospheric legacy in an explicit and systematic manner, despite having made use of it for an extended period.[24] Some authors have tracked its evolutive path, attesting to a beginning a very long time ago. Among these is the architectural historian Alberto Pérez-Gómez, appreciated for his phenomenological approach,[25] who attributes the roots of atmospheric source (in his case: *armonía* and *temperantia*) to Vitruvian thought.

> For Vitruvius harmony is the fundamental quality of beauty (*venustas*), literally sexual attraction: an arrangement of parts that seduces the user/observer and creates a significant, "well-tuned" space for human activities, *the right atmosphere*, in turn, leading to a wholesome, healthy, and meaningful life. (Pérez-Gómez 2016, 43: original italics)

Vitruvius never directly mentions "atmosphere," given that the expression was coined over sixteen hundred years later (to indicate, in technical terms, the mass of air surrounding a celestial body) and would only be used in a figurative sense from the nineteenth century;[26] indeed the word "atmosphere" is only linked to Vitruvius' work in nineteenth-century translations onwards. The *well-tuned space* commented on by Alberto Pérez-Gómez seems to evoke, first and foremost, the vestal, domestic, and social atmosphere that, generated around the hearth, "originally gave rise to the coming together of men, to the deliberative assembly, and to social intercourse" (Vitruvius [first century BC] 1914, book II, chapter I, 38).[27] Such a condition of inclusion and atmospheric contact becomes for Vitruvius, "the origin of the dwelling house."

Thanks to the malleability that marks it out, over time the atmospheric notion acquires an absolute value, becoming "a universally recognized phenomenon that transcends eras and cultures" (Martin 2015, 44). The

---

24 As Barbara Stec notes, "the atmosphere of architecture is not a new phenomenon, but rather a new name for a matter that has existed within architecture since its inception" (2020, 9).
25 See Holl, Pallasmaa, and Pérez-Gómez 1994; Pérez-Gómez 2002.
26 See chapter II "Roots."
27 Vitruvius. 1914. *The Ten Books on Architecture*. Trans. by M.H. Morgan. Cambridge, MA: Harvard University Press (HUP).

atmospheric theme has always been present — in the background — in architectural debate, often appearing in texts and conversations, in both declared and implied forms. Although so familiar, atmosphere is scarcely comparable to other qualities of architectonic space, since "being immersed in atmosphere is an experiential encounter like no other" (Wagenfeld 2015a, 14). This observation, which goes some way to justifying the prolonged period of speculative inertia that has anaesthetized atmospheric reflection in architecture, until the current phase of awakening began at the beginning of the twenty-first century,[28] introduces the eighth point in the analysis of the ineffability of atmosphere: its metaphorical nature.

Eighth unknown: allusiveness

Atmosphere favours allusion with respect to direct and exact expression. In general, it will tend to metaphor. As we have seen, the atmospheric dynamic is not easy to circumscribe and communicate on a verbal plane. For an architect, linguistic expedients — such as metaphors — can help to explain the ambiguities and subtleties that connote the expressive-atmospheric qualities of spaces.[29] As the architectural historian Adrian Forty notes, "language has for the last two hundred years been an ever-open quarry, to which, as new strata become exposed, architects and critics have returned repeatedly to find fresh metaphors" (2000, 64).

Even if architecture is not a language, it does not lessen the value of language as a metaphor for talking about architecture. There is no reason why a metaphor should be required to reproduce every detail of the object to which it is compared: metaphors are never more than partial descriptions of the phenomena they seek to describe, they are always incomplete. Indeed, were they to succeed in total reproduction, they would cease to be metaphors. (Forty 2000, 84)

The use of metaphorical simulation (and its consequent interpretative malleability) becomes advantageous in particular when there is a shift of paradigm from the physical to the mental space. All the more when personal meanings come into play (whether affective, intellective, or cultural), the atmospheric field cannot be classified as a collection of

---

28   See chapter IV "Atmospheric Revival."
29   "Metaphor, rather than being solely a linguistic or rhetorical trope, constitutes a human process by which we understand and structure one domain of experience in terms of another of a different kind" (Johnson 1987 cited in Frampton 1995, 11).

neutral, homogenous, and isotropic qualities, like those that are usually associated with Euclidean space.[30] The atmospheric field is a phenomenal reality (namely, reality as we experience it): it cannot be studied according to a mathematical model, determinable in an axiomatic manner, as could "a space without transcendence, positive, a network of straight lines, parallel among themselves or perpendicular according to the three dimensions" (Merleau-Ponty 1968, 210). On the contrary, atmosphere is space that is "not geometric but lived and pre-dimensional" (Griffero 2020a, 4). In the same way as the notion of *hodological space*,[31] introduced by the psychologist Kurt Lewin (1938) and improved on by the philosopher Otto Friedrich Bollnow ([1963] 2020), it is not possible to predetermine atmospheric space because, depending on lived experience (which is to say, on movements, choices, and the relationships this entails), it can only be expressed extemporaneously as one moves — or, more simply, as one is — in space.

Metaphoric language becomes the liaison between the real world (exterior and material) and the mental world (interior and abstract), capable of evoking the universe of human emotions through the description of the atmospheric qualities attributed to an environment. Although atmospheres cannot properly be considered metaphors (Griffero 2010; Böhme 2013a), for the architectural discipline metaphoric projection of the atmospheric event is a vital approach, from a point of view of both theory and design. Indeed, not only does it provide a valid support as "a lexicalization corrective to otherwise insuperable linguistic deficits" (Griffero 2010, 123), but also it becomes an operative instrument to work with atmospheres. This takes place not so much on a level of constructed metaphors, or rather making use of the metaphor to create scenically atmospheric architecture, as on a level of linguistic metaphor, which is to say adopting the metaphor in the conceptual interpretation of the atmospheric process.

---

30 Maurice Merleau-Ponty, probably the most influential exponent of French phenomenology in the twentieth century, describes Euclidean space as "indifferent to its contents" ([1945] 2002, 63).
31 "Coming from the Greek word ὁδός, a path, it denotes the space opened up by paths [...]. This hodological space is from the start contrasted with abstract mathematical space. [...] Hodological space on the other hand means the change that in concretely lived and experienced space is added to what we had already designated the accessibility of the respective spatial destinations" (Bollnow [1963] 2020, 222–223).

5. Atmospheric Phenomenographies

We have established that atmosphere is extremely difficult (if not impossible) to define, but this does not belie the urgent need to do so. The architect's job is to monitor, transform, and rationalise every aspect of a space, even venturing into the generation of atmospheres. In designing a living space, architecture does not only address shapes, volumes, and solid bodies, it constantly relates to voids too — the arena in which atmospheres manifest themselves. "Men inhabit invisible air and not visible walls," points out Philippe Rahm, the meteorological architect of contemporaneity.[32] "The purpose of architecture is the void space we enter and not inaccessible walls" (2020, 25).

The search for a definition, in the first place semantic, responds to the need to acquire a critical and aware knowledge of the atmospheric question. We have tried to ascertain its limits and potential, without overestimating or skewing the real value of the notion, as there is a propensity to do today (Leatherbarrow 2015). A tension emerges and progressively grows between the apparent non-rationality of the atmospheric theme and the determination to want to comprehend, experiment, represent, and design it (Rauh 2018). Architects intuit that an atmospheric power exists and remain fascinated by it, despite not fully understanding the mechanisms at its base (or, perhaps, precisely because they don't understand them). On the one hand, architects show an increasingly intense interest in the study of atmosphere (Stec 2020), as well as the meaning and function of all those not exclusively visual sensations that enliven the body of architecture;[33] on the other hand, these qualities — ephemeral and immaterial — of our built surroundings put up resistance to the traditional methods of scrutiny and discussion of the spatial experience. They require a more subjective approach, "non-separating" as it were, not detached from the sensory, perceptual, and cognitive capacities of the individual who is living that particular experience.

A possible strategy, to gather and communicate atmospheric impressions, is to *proceed by degrees of intimacy*, progressively less internal and direct

---

32   Philippe Rahm (Lausanne, 1967) heads studio Philippe Rahm Architectes, based in Paris. His work extends the field of architecture into the dimensions of physiology and meteorology.

33   See Neutra 1954; Norberg-Schulz 1971; Bloomer and Moore 1977; Eisenman 1992; Pallasmaa 2002, 2012a; Lupton and Lipps 2018; Robinson 2021.

(Canepa 2021). Option number one, the most anchored to a subjective interpretation of reality, consists in outlining first-person accounts or plotting emotional maps (Bruno 2002), if need be after being lost along unplanned journeys of situationist inspiration (Debord 1958); alternatively, one's own experience could be recorded by an external observer, with recourse to interviews or using quantitative methods aimed at analysing the responses — psychological and/or (neuro)physiological — that the single individual gives in relation to the architectural characteristics of their surroundings;[34] and finally, one might prefer third-person accounts, choosing to adopt an enlarged and objectivising perspective, sometimes intentionally manipulated. In this last case, we incur the risk of producing and conveying standardised visions, which accompany distorted and stereotyped slogans. When we refer to the atmospheric charm of a city, for example, we allude for the most part to a pre-packaged image, so accessible and powerful as to be easily circulated in the globalised market (Griffero 2013).

By a phenomenographic approach, we mean the attempt to describe, at least partially, a phenomenon (in this case, the atmospheric phenomenon) through the point of view of the individual experiencing it.[35] Hence, *atmospheric phenomenography* is the operation of clarifying atmospheric phenomenon by means of one's own subjective and emotional experience. This exercise helps to understand and interpret, in a necessarily deferred way, the atmospheric suggestions that, either due to their imperceptible delicacy or their disruptive force, might have been left undefined at the moment of spatial contact. There is a plurality of possible phenomenographic practices to express the direct experience that we have of a space (De Matteis et al. 2019). For example, there is great atmospheric potential in images (regardless of whether painting, photo, or sketch) to reproduce — but also re-elaborate — the sensation of something experienced.

---

34 It is not just a question of measuring how the experience was consciously lived by the subject (who can describe it, for example, by answering a self-assessment questionnaire), but also of monitoring their corporeal reactions (and therefore, non-verbal, involuntary, and not easily controllable) to the stimuli of the surroundings perceived, as indeed correlated cerebral activity.

35 The term "phenomenography" came into being in the seventies, with the research of the Swedish educational psychologist Ference Marton. "It is research which aims at description, analysis, and understanding of experiences; that is, research which is directed towards experiential description" (1981, 180). Phenomenographic orientation engages as much with experiential as with conceptual aspects, as well as those culturally learned and socially developed.

A Definition Lacking Definition

In the enthusiasm of describing atmospheric sensations, architects have often relied on the expedient of the drawing, to sketch what declinations that words — with their more precise and formalized character — are not able to synthesize. Drawings sit alongside verbal labels, on the basis that "the experience of the drawing is a metaphor of the experience of the building and as such it would be expected to emit something of the ambience of the space" (Karandinou 2013, 23). Even when drawing initial plans, for example, the architect is identifying with the hypothetical user and in their absence simulating, in their own imagination, the montage of situations that will be lived there, the actions that will be carried out, and the physical-sensory sensations that will be perceived. In order to do this, "the laws of experience must be obeyed," warns Le Corbusier. "Man must consider the result in advance" (1929 as reprinted in 2013, 92).

In the drawings (whether rapid studio sketches or sophisticated rendered photomontages), the search for atmospheric effects spills over onto a double plane: on the one side, it permeates the modelling of the architectonic object, to make sure that the general atmosphere resonating through the work transpires in its final configuration (as though it were the most important repercussion of the entire design operation); on the other side, it acts on the aggrandizement of the climatic-environmental conditions, both internal and external, in which the emotional mood of the setting is mirrored. It is no coincidence that most of the time the building is shown at sunset, or standing out against a crystal clear sky, or again, softened within a composition of sparkles and haloes glazing the sketched surfaces. After all, "good architecture is associated with good weather," notes Mark Wigley teasingly (1998a, 20).

So far, without doubt, architectural research into the phenomenon of atmosphere has entrusted more to the analytical and communicative resources of the drawing — although often in forms not fully controlled and informed — than to the elaboration of autonomous theories. What is more, such an approach seems inevitable because, as Professor Wigley notes, "every small choice of representational technique defines an atmosphere" (1998a, 27).

> After all, a drawing is nothing but a decorative surface that exudes an atmosphere like any other surface. The viewer of the drawing is meant to experience something of the building's atmosphere. Drawings are atmosphere simulators and even the most abstract lines produce sensuous, unpredictable effects. (Wigley 1998a, 27)

Nevertheless, there is obviously a leap, a discrepancy, between the graphical rendering of a place and the effective spatial experience that one can undergo in reality, namely in the tangible reproduction of the sketch. However, the complex ineffability that structures atmospheric matter does not seem to be an obstacle even to the repeated attempts, by architects, to integrate it in the construction process. Indeed, among architects, "air, sound, light, fragrance, warmth, smell and other sensory streams are [...] becoming the focus of the creative and experimental endeavor," in addition to "debate and theory-building" (Thibaud 2014a, 49). The words of the artisan-architect Peter Zumthor confirm this incessant quest to educate in the atmospheric sensibility, on a strictly operative level as well.

> Sensing the atmosphere is not so easy at all. It often comes with difficulties. And building the atmosphere, the one that we want, is even more difficult. [laughter] I think that this combination of ideas, moods and emotions with the physical properties of materials, their weight, warmth, hardness, softness, humidity, is very important. It is obvious that, when you take two materials and put them together, you create something between them, some energy. You put them close to each other and see that there is an approximation point at which they begin to interact. Beforehand, they are indifferent, then they connect, but tension arises between the indifference and the connection. The energy, tension and vibrations, the harmony between materials — this is what architecture is to me. (Stec 2004, 90)

6. Seeds

In short: 1. — atmosphere shies away from analysis; 2. — the basic reasons for its indeterminacy are numerous, intrinsically correlated to each other, and hard to interpret; 3. — interest in atmosphere has re-awakened over roughly the last two decades; 4. — architectural culture has entered the interdisciplinary debate, initially reacting with a certain delay compared to other fields of study, which were already occupied with the role of atmosphere in architecture and urban planning;[36] 5. — this book

---

36 The case of the volume *Architecture and Atmosphere* is emblematic, being one of the first publications that declaredly addressed the question of atmosphere in architecture. Published in 2014 (when the "atmospheric turn" is in full swing), it involves four key figures with academic experience around atmosphere: Gernot Böhme, Tonino Griffero, Jean-Paul Thibaud, and Juhani Pallasmaa. Only the last is of purely architectural extraction: the others are, in order, two philosophers and a sociologist. See Tidwell 2014.

will explore the concept of atmosphere from a connotatively architectural point of view, seen in an emotional-sensory perspective, to wit, tied to the properties of the space and direct experience of the subject immersed in the space; 6. — to stem its vague and widespread content, we begin by registering a semantic definition helpful to scientific research of an architectural stamp (and not only).

"Atmosphere" is meant to be a (more) ordered word to perceive and understand, although the ambiguity shrouding it up to the present day has been useful to its vitality. It is thought that a greater clarity would facilitate a more authoritative and informed debut, in the architectural dialectic, setting out from its hoped-for acceptance by dictionaries and manuals in the sector, which until now have shown a dearth of entries.[37] The need for a verified definition goes beyond a presumed neurosis of diachrony, of cultural mores. Although it is undeniable that "like any other social phenomenon, architecture reflects fads and fashions" (Borch 2014, 7), the (new) appeal of atmospheric aesthetics deserves deep analysis, which does not reduce the scope of the event to a voluble tendency of the present moment. Placed in the correct historical perspective, continuity and stability can be seen to be growing constantly. What is needed is *a contemporary architectural definition* that can absorb the legacies of the past and integrate new insights of critical resonance, like those issuing from a comparison with modern cognitive neuroscience. The operation performed is meant to be an experiment, an incipit. As Fernando Espuelas states in his fine book on the empty space, accepted as resource and project vision alike, "a desirable fate for this essay would be for it to transform, in the manner of a palimpsest, into a base on which to accumulate future contributions [...] to be a seed rather than a scythe" (1999, 10). From atmospheric seed, the first to push up shoots were the numerous, or rather innumerable, emergent queries. Some have found an answer; others continue to flutter over the path of newly charted research.

---

[37] Notes on the concept of atmosphere — in encyclopaedic contexts relevant to the architectural discipline — are currently to be found in De Matteis 2020 (s.v. "Atmosphere in Architecture," n.p.); Gregory 2020 (s.v. "Atmosfera," 115–119); Pallasmaa and Zambelli 2020 (s.vv. "Atmospheres in Architecture," 28–31; "Atmospheric Intelligence," 31–32; "Atmospheres in the Arts," 32–33; "Atmospheric Sense [the]," 34–35). In passing: the entry "Atmosphere (Architecture and Spatial Design)" is described on Wikipedia, the famous online encyclopaedia with freely edited content. The architectural meaning was the first contribution to deal with the theme of atmosphere on a figurative level, that is, not tied to the technical definition of gaseous mass.

Le Corbusier had a point. Throughout his career he had a conflictual relationship with atmospheric effects, unable to subjugate them to the forces of pure and rational objectification (Pérez-Gómez 2016, 18): picking up a *thick notebook* would be useful to note down all the doubts and tack together the various hypotheses of a solution.

II
ROOTS

1. Semantic Geography

Atmosphere
noun —[1]

1. (literal sense)
a. The spheroidal gaseous envelope surrounding any of the heavenly bodies.
b. Specially: the mass of aeriform fluid surrounding the earth; the whole body of terrestrial air.

2. (transferred sense)
A gaseous envelope surrounding any substance.

3. (obsolete)
a. A supposed outer envelope of effective influence surrounding various bodies; especially: *electrical atmosphere*, that surrounding electrified bodies.
b. *Magnetic atmosphere*, the sphere within which the attractive force of the magnet acts.

4. (figurative sense)
a. Surrounding mental or moral element, environment. Also, prevailing psychological climate; pervading tone or mood; characteristic mental or moral environment; fascinating or beguiling associations or effects.
b. Specially: applied to the background sounds that evoke a particular mood, impression, setting, etc., in a broadcast programme, etc.

5. (air)
The air in any particular place, especially as affected in its condition by heat, cold, purifying or contaminating influences, etc.

6. (atmospheric pressure)
A pressure of 15 lbs. on the square inch, which is that exerted by the atmosphere on the earth's surface.

---

[1] "Atmosphere," in *The Oxford English Dictionary*. 2nd edn, 1989. Prepared by J.A. Simpson and E.S.C. Weine, vol. I, 750. Oxford: Clarendon Press.

A rapid glance at the term "atmosphere" in any dictionary[2] is enough to become aware of the jagged nature of atmosphere's semantic geography: it is run through with a thick network of roots that spread out towards compound horizons of meaning, both technical and figurative.

2. Genesis

The etymology of the word "atmosphere"[3] is based on the Indo-European root *au-t* (transposition of *ua-t* or *va-t*), which means "to blow." This primary nucleus reappears in the Greek ἀτμός (*atmos*), translatable as "vapour," "air," or "breath;" there follows the combination with the noun σφαῖρα (*sphaira*), literally "sphere," "globe," or "ball" — from which derives the expression currently used to indicate the mass of gaseous fluid enveloping a planet or, in general, any celestial body with a somewhat intense gravitational field. The compound lemma (ἀτμός + σφαῖρα), produced by two Greek language words, instinctively evokes a classical lineage; but that is not the case: it is a Greek neologism (Spitzer 1942b), which came into being in the modern era and progressively spread through the European linguistic systems,[4] that doesn't belong to the (ancient) Greek[5]

---

2 The reconstruction of the genesis and historical evolution of the term "atmosphere" was originally focused, in the author's doctoral dissertation (Canepa 2019), above all on the Italian language context, of which it lacked a systematic study. This is the reason why some of the next references are specific to the Italian linguistic legacy. Nonetheless, they can be read as fragments of an ampler and more transversal process, shared, as far as can be seen, in other European languages. For example, for a comparison with German and its literary culture, see Spitzer 1942a, 1942b; Riedel 2019.

3 "Atmosphere," in *An Etymological Dictionary of Modern English*. 1921. Ed. by E. Weekley, 86. London: John Murray.

4 DE: *atmosphäre* (f.); EN: *atmosphere* (f.); ES: *atmósfera* (f.); FR: *atmosphère* (f.); IT: *atmosfera* (f.); NL: (*atmo*)*sfeer* (f.); PT: *atmosfera* (f.); RO: *atmosferă* (f.).

5 We find straightforward proof of this by consulting a dictionary of ancient Greek, where the term ατμόσφαιρα is not present. See *Gl: Vocabolario della Lingua Greca*. 1995. Ed. by F. Montanari. Torino: Loescher. Instead, the lemma was absorbed by the evolution of modern Greek, both by its literary and figurative acceptation. See *English Greek Dictionary*. 1997. English-Greek section (45). Glasgow: HarperCollins.
    As presented by the Austrian linguist and literary critic Leo Spitzer (1887–1960) in his detailed semantic analysis of words that unite to define the concept of atmosphere, "we find in Greek ὁ περιέχων ἀήρ or τὸ περιέχον, an expression meaning literally 'that which surrounds, encompasses' (from the verb περι-έχειν), and used to refer to the all-embracing air, space, sky, atmosphere, climate" (1942a, 2).

or the Latin[6] lexical repertoire. A semantic path by no means anomalous, and similar to that of other lexemes in the modern register.[7]

The Latin form *atmosphaera* began to circulate in Europe from the middle of the seventeenth century (Martin 2015), initially appearing in the writings of cosmologists and meteorologists, and later, towards the end of the century, in botanical and medical treatises.[8] It was the Flemish astronomer and mathematician Willebrord Snellius (1580–1626)[9] who first introduced the noun in 1608: he edited the Latin translation of the essays on cosmography published in those years by his compatriot Simon Stevin (1548–1620),[10] physicist and engineer who, convinced of the superiority of the Dutch language in scientific communication, rejected the Latin and, to synthesize the image of a sphere of vapour, coined the compound word *dampcloot*.[11] From that moment, the neologism *atmosphaera* was known and adopted by numerous intellectuals of the period: among them Snellius himself, who made use of it in his treatise on the comets of 1619.[12] The *Oxford English Dictionary* attributes the first use of the term in a work drafted in English (1638)[13] to the Anglican clergyman and natural

---

6 As in the previous case, we consulted a Latin dictionary, where no entry for *atmosphaera* is included. See *Cassell's Latin Dictionary*. 1953. Rev. by J.R.V. Marchant and J.F. Charles. New York, NY: Funk and Wagnalls. In the English-Latin section (645), the word "atmosphere" is translated as *caelum* with a suggested link to the entry "air."
7 Two more famous examples are the words "nostalgia" (a condensation of νόστος — "return" and άλγος — "pain," "sadness") and "aesthetic" (resulting from the matrix αἴσθησις — "sensation," "perception"): the first was invented in the seventeenth century by an Alsatian medical student at the University of Basel, Johannes Hofer (1669–1752); the second was coined in the eighteenth century by the German philosopher Alexander Gottlieb Baumgarten (1714–1762).
8 In the field of medicine, the idea that atmosphere, as the air that human beings breathe, had an active influence on their health and physical constitution was already upheld by Hippocrates in the fifth century BC (Spitzer 1942a; Leatherbarrow 2015).
9 It is to Willebrord Snellius, better known in the English-speaking world simply as Snell, that the law of refraction of light is attributed.
10 Stevin, Simon. 1608. "Secunda Pars Cosmographiae: De Geographia." In *Hypomnemata Mathematica* (1605–1608), trans. by W. Snellius. Lugduni Batavorum (Leiden): Ex Officina Ioannis Patii, Academiae Typographi.
11 Literal translation: "vapour-ball."
12 Snellius, Willebrord. 1619. *Descriptio Cometæ*. Lugduni Batavorum (Leiden): Ex Officina Elzeviriana.
13 Wilkins, John. 1638. *The Discovery of a World in the Moone: Or a Discourse Tending to Prove That 'tis Probable There May Be Another Habitable World in*

philosopher John Wilkins (1614–1672). The Latin loanword was initially used to describe the thick layer of gas, that was assumed to encompass the moon; it is odd to note that the first appearance of the word "atmosphere" is connected to the moon, which today has been demonstrated to lack an effective atmospheric shield: earth's natural satellite is surrounded by a veil so thin and unstable in density as to be equated to the void.

The neologism "atmosphere" takes its place in Italian scientific literature with a few years' delay: approximately around 1667.[14] It is the Florentine erudite Lorenzo Magalotti (1637–1712) who imported the word,[15] including it in the lines of the letter entitled *Sopra la Luce* (Above the Light), which he sent to his master Vincenzo Viviani. The missive is not dated, but was certainly written before 1667, the year that the Accademia del Cimento (the Academy of Experiment) was dissolved and his diplomatic activity abroad began.

Very quickly, as Friedlind Riedel (2020) clearly highlights, the proto-scientific concept of atmosphere spreads into the medical and pharmaceutical languages too. We can identify two fundamental primary strands of meaning: on the one side, a meaning of meteorological origin, from which comes "atmosphere as ambient air," or rather "the sphere surrounding celestial bodies," and "the pneumatic substance of life;" on the other side, a meaning of bodily origin, from which derives the concept of "atmosphere as effluvia," or initially as an exhalation of odours and aromas, then as "the aerial, elastic, magnetic or electric effluvia that emanated from and enveloped the human body" (Riedel, 9–10). The main difference between the two interpretations is that the idea of *atmosphere as ambient air* is, by its very nature, lacking a nucleus and a precise spatialization, while the premise of *atmosphere as effluvia* necessarily implies the presence of a material source that produces it.

That Planet. London: E.G. for Michael Sparke and Edward Forrest. — "*That there is an Atmo-sphæra, or an orbe of grosse vaporous aire, immediately encompassing the body of the Moone*" (138: original italics).

14 "Atmosfera," in *Dizionario Etimologico della Lingua Italiana (DELI)*. 2nd edn, 1999. Ed. by M. Cortelazzo and M.A. Cortelazzo, 142. Bologna: Zanichelli.

15 An interesting etymological reconstruction of the entry "atmosfera," recognising Magalotti for the first use of the neologism in a work edited in Italian, is illustrated in Turolo, Antonio. 1994. *Tradizione e rinnovamento nella lingua delle "Lettere scientifiche ed erudite" del Magalotti*. Firenze: Accademia della Crusca.

3. Metaphorical Inversion

Whilst over the years the proto-scientific sense of the concept of atmosphere prospers and matures, in other words a pre-eminently physical meaning that is describable and tends to be measurable, a second connotation emerges, which before long acquires significant autonomy. In the course of the nineteenth century, a figurative sense germinates and is assimilated to distinguish — in allusive tones — the emotional, psychological, or moral sphere of influence of a particular ambience. According to the extended definition given in the *Oxford English Dictionary*, the first figurative use of the term dates back to the start of the nineteenth century.[16] There follows a long literary tradition, counting among its forerunners the English poet Samuel Taylor Coleridge (1772–1834).[17]

Over the same decades, the Italian cultural engine begins to interpret the atmospheric lexical unit metaphorically: the *Grande Dizionario della Lingua Italiana* by Salvatore Battaglia outlines the period of incubation through a broad set of examples. Beginning with a text by the Renaissance poet Giuseppe Giusti (1809–1850) from 1839,[18] it touches on a wide list of authors, increasing in modernity; such as Giovanni Verga, Ferdinando Paolieri, Ignazio Silone, Alberto Moravia, and Cesare Pavese. The evolution of the meaning has its origin in the absorption of the French form *atmosphère*,[19] adopted in 1787: the calque and its consequent allusive turn

---

16 1797–1803: Foster, John. *Life and Corr.*, I. 163. — "An extensive atmosphere of Consciousness."
17 Coleridge, Samuel T. 1847. *Biographia Literaria: Or, Biographical Sketches of My Literary Life and Opinions*. 2nd edn. Prepared for publication in part by the late H.N. Coleridge, completed and published by his widow. London: William Pickering. First published: 1817. London: Rest Fenner. — "It was the union of deep feeling with profound thought; the fine balance of truth in observing, with the imaginative faculty in modifying, the objects observed; and above all the original gift of spreading the tone, the atmosphere, and with it the depth and height of the ideal world around forms, incidents, and situations, of which, for the common view, custom had bedimmed all the lustre, had dried up the sparkle and the dew drops" (79).
18 Giusti, Giuseppe. 1939. "Lettera a Silvio Giannini." In *Epistolario*, ordered by G. Frassi. Firenze: Felice Le Monnier. — "A trent'anni chi non è stato chiuso ermeticamente in un'atmosfera di beata melensaggine, pur troppo sente d'aver perdute tutte le illusioni" (vol. I, 185).
19 "Atmosphère," in *Le Grand Robert de la Langue Française*. 2nd edn, 2001. Ed. by A. Rey, 926–927. Paris: Dictionnaires Le Robert. The neologism is documented for the first time in 1665 (Chapelain, Jean. *Lettre adressée à Pierre-Daniel Huet*),

are severely frowned on by late nineteenth century purists.[20] For example, philologists Pietro Fanfani (1815–1879) and Costantino Arlìa (1829–1915) include the word *atmosfera* in the list of Gallicisms that fatten the lexicon of the lowly and corrupted Italian spirit, and suggest it be substituted by a more integral synonym, such as "state."[21] In the same period Giuseppe Rigutini (1829–1903) holds a less intransigent position with regard to purist lexicography; however, not even he relinquishes contesting the new figurative spoken uses, to which the word "atmosphere"[22] adheres.

Despite an initial approach of diffidence and the obstinate attempts to stem its spread, the loan word experiences an ample and widespread diffusion, to the extent that today, in its figurative meaning, it is considered a component of *common* use Italian, even distinguishing itself as a *fundamental* unit in the case of the extended meaning of "the air we breathe."[23]

---

while its metaphorical inflexion is thought to have appeared in the eighteenth century.

20   "Atmosfera," in *Dizionario Etimologico della Lingua Italiana (DELI)*. 2nd edn, 1999. Ed. by M. Cortelazzo and M.A. Cortelazzo, 142. Bologna: Zanichelli.

21   "Atmosfera," in *Lessico dell'Infima e Corrotta Italianità*. 3rd edn, 1890. Ed. by P. Fanfani and C. Arlìa, 49. Milano: Paolo Carrara. — "È un'eleganza per taluni il dire, p.e.: *Le cose politiche ci fanno vivere in un'atmosfera d'incertezza* [...] Regolatamente puoi usare 'stato;' così nell'esempio: *Le cose politiche ci fanno vivere in uno stato d'incertezza*" (original italics).

22   "Atmosfera," in *I Neologismi Buoni e Cattivi più Frequenti nell'Uso Odierno*. 1886. Ed. by G. Rigutini, 122. Roma: Carlo Verdesi. — "Anche questa è una delle voci del linguaggio fisico, di cui oggi si abusa a significare cose morali: *Atmosfera di odj, di vizj; Vivere in una serena atmosfera; La calma atmosfera di una conversazione; I giovani oggi respirano un'atmosfera di corruzione*, e cento altre di queste atmosfere, prese con tanti altri parlari figurati dai nostri vicini" (original italics).

23   "Atmosfera," in *Grande Dizionario Italiano dell'Uso*. 1999. Ed. by T. De Mauro, vol. I, 482–483. Torino: Unione Tipografico-Editrice Torinese (UTET). The term is listed in the *fundamental lexicon* family, which constitutes the nucleus of the language's most important lexemes: slightly more than two thousand words, of very high-frequency use, which alone cover about 90% of the lexical instances in text and discourse. Noteworthy, however, is that the figurative meaning is listed as *common*, or as a lemma used and understood independently of profession or occupation, or regional location, and generally known to anyone with an average education. The word "atmosphere" has not undergone a decline in use, as can be seen in the *Nuovo Vocabolario di Base della Lingua Italiana*. 2016. Ed. by T. De Mauro — online at *Internazionale* (www.internazionale.it, last accessed 17 October 2021).

In the season of Romanticism, the term takes on new cultural inflexions, imposing itself as a semantic vehicle to describe inter-subjective relations of varied types (among which social, psychological, sentimental, and ethical), between two or more individuals as well as the surroundings — natural or humanised — in which they are immersed. Atmospheres become "sensory structures of communicable feeling, at once somatic and ideal, aesthetic and material, affective and conceptual" (Ford 2018, 20). Reaching such a state of evolution has taken a long series of steps (Riedel 2019, 2020), which involve both the meteorological vein of significance and that of corporeal inspiration.

Over the years, the meteorological sense of the concept of atmosphere gains a progressively more collective and enlarged dimension, "mobilised as metaphor to refer to the intellectual and spiritual, but also moral, environments" (Riedel 2020, 9). By taking this trajectory we reach, for example, the aesthetics vision of Gernot Böhme, who explicitly states that the term "atmosphere" derives from meteorological science.

> The term *atmosphere* was originally used within meteorological contexts. Here it designated the upper part of the air mantling the earth. But since the eighteenth century *atmosphere* was used as metaphor describing a certain mood hanging in the air. The mediating link obviously is the weather: the weather is affecting my mood — a rising thunderstorm may frighten me, bright weather may raise my spirits. Today atmosphere may be defined briefly as *tuned space*, i.e. a space with a certain mood. (Böhme 2017c, 2: original italics)

The second strand of meaning, however, referring to the idea of corporeal effluvia, endorses a more individual reading, which from emanating material (sensorially perceptible in the first place through the sense of smell) extends to the sphere of corporeal conditions, sentiments, and lived experiences. "Since emanations varied according to gender, occupation, diet, and habitat," explains Friedlind Riedel, taking inspiration from the French historian Alain Corbin (1986), "atmospheres were social indicators, suggestive of the character of a person, their social class, and emotional situation" (2019, 86–87).

With the passing of time, some inflexions have declined (among which, for example, the use of "atmosphere" as a medical expression, the vehicle for propagating contagious illnesses, such as cholera), while others have reinforced and evolved.[24] At present, contamination — between literal reference and figurative allusion — is complete, intrinsically imbued with an unexpected and innovative potential; namely, its flexible character, an elegant balance between specialist and indefinite, consigning the noun to a process of dispersion among different genres of knowledge. Each of these re-elaborates the meaning, moving within its disciplinary context.

4. Detonation

A branched palimpsest of semantic nuances has gradually grafted onto the primitive root of the term "atmosphere," loaned to fields of enquiry that are very different from each other, to address both technical questions and instances of an affective slant.

In *physics*, the study of atmosphere — in the meaning of gaseous mass — mixes the analysis of its chemical-physical composition with the design of the universe's limits.

In *meteorology*, earthly atmosphere is monitored by means of the observation of the natural phenomena that agitate and that have an effect on the climate (such as clouds, wind, and rain).

In *metrology*, atmosphere is converted into a standard unit of pressure (symbol: atm): much employed in the past, although today substituted in the international system by Pascal (symbol: Pa), its use is still frequently adopted in everyday language.

In *acoustics*, atmosphere is defined as "the noise deliberately introduced into a recording or broadcast to disguise an unnaturally silent interval."[25]

In the *applied sciences*, in general, special conditions are experimented with, interpolating the physical, chemical, molecular, and electrical

---

24 For example, there is a very original interpretation formulated by the Australian-American philosopher Teresa Brennan (1952–2003), for whom atmospheric contact acts also on the individual at a biochemical and physiological level. Brennan specifically focuses on the role pheromone odours play in the ways in which an atmosphere is perceived and affection is transmitted. See Brennan 2004.
25 "Atmosphere," in *Sound: International Dictionary*. 1975 (47). Milano: Franco Angeli.

properties of the atmospheric fluid: in this way, atmospheres are generated that are controlled, normal, standard, and universal.[26]

In *law*, atmosphere asserts its physical corporeality: juridical discipline sees the theory of the freedom of atmosphere contrast with the theory of sovereignty, in the attempt to regulate air traffic and radio communications polity.

In *social sciences*, in the wide sense, atmosphere reflects the socio-environmental identity of a group or of a context in which social experiences happen that are crucial for the individual. In particular, talking of urban spaces, atmosphere is considered by some scholars to be a sort of "skin" (Hasse 2014), which becomes an indicator of the social conditions that characterise the city and of the perceptual rejects tied to its image.

In *philosophy*, atmospheric research (which was the object of much study in the first half of the twentieth century and has now returned to the limelight) is part of the age-old debate on spatial experiences, aimed at finding an interpretation that can go beyond a merely physical-geometric reading of our surroundings. Atmospheres, according to an approach that is mainly inspired by Neue Ästhetik (Gernot Böhme) and Neue Phänomenologie (Hermann Schmitz), are specific qualities of a particular *lived space*, to wit the space in which the *felt body* moves and experiences.[27]

In *literature*, a narrative approach has developed, exemplified in "atmospheric" novels, where the characters, their state of mind, surroundings, landscape, and the story, almost blending together, create a fused whole: it is no longer individual details that surface, but the all-encompassing entity, in its capacity to trigger emotional vibrations.

In *cinema* and *theatre*, the atmosphere genre imitates the expressive mechanisms consolidated in the literary tradition and amplifies their

---

26 The *International Standard Atmosphere* (ISA) was adopted on 7 November 1952 by the International Civil Aviation Organization (ICAO). It defines an ideal model of average actual atmosphere, to use as a reference for purposes such as calibrating altimeters, calculating ballistic tables, or designing aircraft and missiles.
27 For further information on the (philosophical) history of the concept of *lived space* (from Martin Heidegger to Hermann Schmitz), see Griffero 2014b.

suggestions, resounding around the scenographic system. The spectator is involved in the flow of indeterminacy and urged to supply with their imagination what has been deliberately left vague, as in an act of creative catharsis.

In the field of *music*, the particular acoustic and atmospheric qualities of a place find the correct tuning in "ambient music," whose properties were specified by the person considered to be its inventor, the British composer Brian Eno: "an ambience is defined as an atmosphere, or a surrounding influence: a tint."[28]

In *art*, atmosphere is the mass of air that envelops bodies and objects and alters their values at a distance: what the Greeks called ἀήρ, the Latins *aër*. Techniques of representation and setting are entrusted to aerial aesthetic principles (such as chiaroscuro and the effects of relief), in which the distance of the point of observation and the specific light, illuminating the scene, shape the plastic-atmospheric sense that connotes the work.

In *architecture*, the notion of atmosphere has assumed the role of compelling centrality in contemporary research and practice, but an explicit delimitation of boundaries of its semantic spectrum is slow to establish itself.

5. Architectural Genealogy

Today it is hard to dismiss the impression that the atmospheric approach has become a core issue for the design practice and for critical understanding of the architectural discipline. However, determining when this ascent began is not easy. With reference to the historical reconstruction put forward by Harry Francis Mallgrave (2018), it is likely that the first architect to make use of the word "atmosphere" — in a text pertinent to the design subject — was the German Gottfried Semper (1803–1879). In 1860, with regard to the use of textile art as a decorative and furnishing element, he wrote this consideration.

---

28   Eno, Brian. 1978. "Ambient Music." Liner notes from the album *Ambient 1: Music for Airports*. UMC Virgin.

Every artistic creation, every artistic pleasure, presumes a certain carnival spirit, or to express it in a modern way, the haze of carnival candles is the true atmosphere [*wahre Atmosphäre*] of art. (Semper 2004, 438–439 n. 85)

Again, according to Mallgrave, at the dawn of the twentieth century the expression "atmosphere" becomes relatively common in various architectural circles: Frank Lloyd Wright (1867–1959), for example, dwells on to the concept on numerous occasions, conscious of its importance (Pallasmaa 2013). "Yet this emotionally laden term all but disappeared in the second half of the century," continues Harry Francis Mallgrave in his reconstruction (2018, 121); it will only rise out of oblivion a few decades later, with the aesthetics revival promoted in particular by Gernot Böhme (1937–2022), "one of the pioneering thinkers in the philosophy of atmospheres" (Pallasmaa 2014a, 233). Personally, I believe that the word "atmosphere" continued to circulate in architects' expressive territory, although often changing appearance (with synonyms and foreign loan words), never framed in a precise and shared sense system. Consulting the *Encyclopedic Dictionary of Architecture and Urban Planning* edited by Paolo Portoghesi (1968),[29] there is no trace of the word to be found, even in its technical-physical inflexion: with nothing between the entry *atlante* ("atlas") and the adjective *atomico* ("atomic"). The same absence is revealed in the Anglophone *A Dictionary of Architecture* (1999) by John Fleming, Hugh Honour, and Nikolaus Pevsner.[30] In more recent dictionaries,[31] some collections (above all among handbooks) carry the lemma, declining it exclusively in applied terms, among which "atm," "atmospheric pressure," "atmospheric layers," "atmospheric projection," "atmospheric burner."

If in manuals and dictionaries, the architectural culture does not seem to be aware of the relevance of the atmospheric concept, it does emerge

---

29 Portoghesi, Paolo (ed.). 1968. *Dizionario Enciclopedico di Architettura e Urbanistica*. Roma: Istituto Editoriale Romano.
30 Fleming, John, Honour, Hugh, and Pevsner, Nikolaus (eds.). 1999. *Dictionary of Architecture and Landscape Architecture* (1966). 5th edn. London: Penguin Books.
31 See Cowan, Henry J., and Smith, Peter R. (eds.). 2004. *Dictionary of Architectural and Building Technology* (1973). 4th edn. London and New York, NY: Spon Press; Harris, Cyril M. (ed.). 2006. *Dictionary of Architecture and Construction* (1975). 4th edn. New York, NY: McGraw-Hill; Davies, Nikolas, and Jokiniemi, Erkki (eds.). 2008. *Dictionary of Architecture and Building Construction*. Oxford and Burlington, MA: Architectural Press, Elsevier.

— with a certain spontaneity — in the language of some architects and is reflected in coeval architecture journals, between which there is inevitable contamination. An episode that confirms this attitude to *lexical symbiosis*, and that witnesses a familiarity — already rooted in time — with the theme of atmosphere, goes back to 1954. Franco Albini (1905–1977), in his inaugural lecture at the University Institute of Architecture of Venice (IUAV)[32] on the topics of art and decoration, stresses the fundamental role of atmospheric suggestion and the importance of staging "atmospheric spaces."

> The inventive exhibition design should engage the visitor in its game; the right atmospheres should be generated around the works to enhance them, but without ever overwhelming them. Architecture should be the mediator between the audience and the things on display, it should give value to the environment as a powerful element for the creation of impressions in the visitor. To achieve this, in my view, one must use spatial rather than plastic solutions: we need to create architectural spaces, to underline existing ones, linking them in absolute unity with the works exhibited. In my opinion what must be constructed is precisely the empty space, as air and light are construction materials. The atmosphere should not be still, stagnant, it should be vibrant, and the viewer should feel immersed and stimulated without noticing what is happening. (Albini 2005, 99)

Federico Bucci, among the leading scholars of Albini's work, observed that however much he simulates a confidential relationship with the aesthetics of atmosphere, it seems "extraneous to the vocabulary of Franco Albini and his figurative world" (2005, 100). Approaching this concept would result from the influence of his friend and colleague Giovanni Romano (1905–1990), who in 1941 drew on the allusive aspect of atmospheric poetics to describe in *Domus* a project of Franco Albini's, which is to say the interior design set up of his private home in Aristide De Togni street, in Milan.[33]

In the full text (heavy with expressions such as "atmospheric volumes" and "atmospheric spaces"), the reference to the expressive quality of atmosphere seems obvious, instinctive, an inherent part of the architectural lexicon. Today, eighty years after Giovanni Romano took the photograph,

---

32 To open the academic year 1954–1955.
33 "An architecture that makes use of atmospheric spaces, bordered only in ideal terms by hints, as of architectural elements, composing them with constructed architectonic elements" (Romano 1941, 15).

the concept of atmosphere, despite not appearing as a permanent definition in architectural dictionaries, runs rampant in the communicative imagination of the design journals[34] and architectural critical reviews. Not needing to respect precise semantic boundaries, the word "atmosphere" sweeps over a vast landscape of interpretations that are accepted and gain a growing autonomy. An example, held symptomatic of this tendency, is given in the column "Meteorology" by Philippe Rahm, which appeared, for the entire year 2018, in the pages of *Domus* edited by Michele De Lucchi. Here, the atmospheric event takes on the role of undisputed protagonist, manifested by the title itself. Rahm decides to clarify the meaning of the atmospheric phenomenon, restricting it to a specific area (an original synthesis of physiology, thermodynamics, and climatology), to raise it to a founding act of the architectural discipline.

> Architecture is basically the design of the atmosphere. [...] Rather than reasoning in terms of grid, structure, symmetry and form, we must learn to reason in terms of convection, conduction, emissivity and effusiveness. Rather than working in brick, concrete, steel or wood, we have to work with light, heat, shade or moisture. (Rahm 2018, 107)

This is just one of the innumerable types of atmosphere recognised in the architectural field. The *Atlas of Atmospheres*, illustrated in the following chapter, tries to piece together the full range. What matters, in this step, is noticing the pressing need with which the reflection on the diachronic development of the lexical element "atmosphere" within the architectural language is put forward. The present-day atmospheric ferment is bubbling on extremely fluid and unstable ground, not only strewn with semantic shifts, but also infused with synonyms and loans from other languages.

---

34 In some cases, entire issues of architecture and design journals have been, recently, dedicated to the theme of atmosphere. For example: *Daidalos. Architecture Art Culture / Architektur Kunst Kultur* 68 (1998): "Constructing Atmospheres / Konstruktion von Atmosphären;" *OASE. Journal for Architecture / Tijdschrift voor architectuur* 91 (2013): "Building Atmosphere / Sfeer bouwen;" *Ambiances. International Journal of Sensory Environment, Architecture and Urban Space* 5 (2019): "Phenomenographies: Describing Urban and Architectural Atmospheres;" *GUD. A Magazine about Architecture, Design and Cities* 2 (2020): "Conclusus;" *VENTI Journal: Air, Experience, and Aesthetics* 1 (2020): "Atmosphere."

6. Thesaurus

From a lexical basis there is still one question to analyse: the disorderly straggle of synonyms, loan words, and adaptations that have settled and accumulated on the lemma "atmosphere," blurring with it. Among the synonyms that cause the literary-figurative sense to increase, more generic expressions abound — such as *air, ambience, environment, spirit, tone*.[35] If we take into consideration the meteorological lineage of the term, and so the designation of atmosphere as an ambient quality, we encounter very common synonyms like *climate, nimbus, aura, fluid*; "and perhaps *emanation* should be counted among them as well" (Böhme 1998, 112). Then there are alternatives that are more coherent with architectural phrasing: *ambiance, lived space, mood, Stimmung, temperament, feeling, attunement*, and *milieu*. Finally, we note more infrequent variants such as *Umwelt* ("ambient" in German), *ki* (Japanese concept that, portraying the steam rising from cooking rice, alludes to the vital spirit that pervades a place), the German *Zwischen*, and its English equivalent *in-between*, all nouns that hide the founding idea of atmospheres; and, that is, their being "a vague ens or power, without visible and discrete boundaries, which we find around us and, resonating in our lived body, even involves us."[36]

This disintegration of stylistic-expressive hues is an added indicator of the difficulty we encounter in defining the noetic field of the linguistic atmospheric code, namely the body of meanings that it allows. The word "atmosphere" has an equivalent in every European language, employable on a literary or figurative level, almost as constant from a graphical point of view.[37] The choice of one variant rather than another depends on the sensitivity of the particular author or, more simply, their expressive habits. The cases below represent only a reduced fraction of the detectable preferences; they belong to highly heterogeneous contexts (both on chronological and geographic-cultural levels), and it cannot be supposed

---

35 "Atmosphere," in *The Oxford Thesaurus: An A–Z Dictionary of Synonyms*. 1991. Ed. by L. Urdang. Oxford: Clarendon Press.
36 Extract from the presentation of the series *Atmospheric Spaces*, edited by Tonino Griffero (Milano and Udine: Mimesis International).
37 The more delicate situation is in German. Although various experts use the term *Atmosphäre* (e.g., Hermann Schmitz and Gernot Böhme), it is the word *Stimmung* (essentially untranslatable) that recreates the full spectrum of suggestions and references that the concept of atmosphere has acquired in other tongues (Spitzer 1942b, 188–189 n. 61).

that they are more significant in an absolute sense. Basically, they provide a sufficiently varied panorama, bringing more detailed references to the abovementioned list of alternative semantics.

The Situationists, for example, making use of French to convey their theoretical output in the pages of the journal *Internationale Situationniste* (1958–1969), adopted the term *ambiance*[38] to describe the emotional potential that pervades a place, namely its atmospheric identity. At the same time, they baptised *unités d'ambiance* those areas of the city, mapped out through the act of *dérive* ("drift"), seen as having a "particularly intense urban atmosphere" (Sadler 1999, 69). Thus *ambiance* — literally translatable as "atmosphere" — assumes the meaning of "totality of material conditions that are essential for the collective construction of a situation," where *situation* is understood as "a mere 'moment de la vie,' in other words, short-lived and intended to be succeeded by new and different situations" (Constant 1998, 232).

In other cases, we see borrowed labels coined in adjacent disciplinary fields: undoubtedly philosophical studies exercise a strong influence, among the first to take on issues of this type. A demonstration is provided by the notion of *tempered space* (in German: *gestimmter Raum*), introduced by certain phenomenologists such as Otto Friedrich Bollnow ([1963] 2020) and Elisabeth Ströker (1965). Whereas Gernot Böhme, who continues that line of research, favours the expression *atmosphere* to that of *tempered space*, maintaining that while the first portrays "the space of mindful physical presence," the second suggests the idea that "the space is assumed to be there as such and then tempered by a specific mood" (2013b, 27). In this way Böhme recalls the terminology used by the main exponent of the Neue Phänomenologie,[39] Hermann Schmitz (1967, 2014, 2016).[40]

The selection of a single noun that condenses the ample range of thoughts might be the most complex aspect of the whole research project. This point is made by Professor Alberto Pérez-Gómez, who prefers not to cite the word "atmosphere" directly to discuss the atmospheric construct in architecture, entitling his book on the subject *Attunement* (2016). He clarifies that "one must understand the concept of atmosphere in light of

---

38   Jean-Paul Thibaud explains the context for the notion of *ambiance* (2015).
39   New Phenomenology, in English. See Schmitz 2019.
40   Hermann Schmitz (1928–2021) can be considered the founder of research into atmospheres in a German-speaking context (Kazig 2016).

the full linguistic range that the German word *Stimmung* possessed [at the] inception" (Pérez-Gómez, 32). The basic idea is that the English (and Italian) "atmosphere" remains an ambiguous semantic vector, not as clear as *Stimmung* in German. Picking up the philological studies of the linguist Leo Spitzer (1963, 6),[41] Pérez-Gómez distils the two prevalent semantic ideas in the *Stimmung* concept that are woven into ancient and medieval thought: the principles of "well-tempered mixture" and "harmonious consonance" (2016, 34).

7. Coagulation

"That's all we have, finally, the words, and they had better be the right ones," Raymond Carver exhorts us to be careful in his essay *On Writing*.[42] Therefore, faced with the vast range of tones of meaning, synonyms, and foreign loan words, this book chooses the expression "atmosphere" to encompass, absorb, and substitute all the alternatives analysed. The decision to uphold this word is tied, above all, to its intrinsic semantic plasticity, which has rendered it to this day an element well infiltrated and settled in common language. Every reference to it is immediate and efficient; it works both in colloquial use and in instances of a scientific-academic nature; it involves as much the members of the architectural community as the layperson; it can be communicated on a local and international scale. The word even holds commercial potential (Kotler 1973), which, recognised at the concept, clarifies and verifies its use adaptability. To give an example: the Scandinavian multinational Ikea, colossus in the sale of furniture and furnishing accessories, has recently invested part of its advertising campaign in the promotion of atmospheric sensitivity. This can be seen in the messages appearing in the pages of their famous catalogue (2018–2021). Atmosphere becomes a resounding slogan.[43]

---

41   Spitzer attributes to the term *Stimmung* the capacity both to formalize an objective understanding of the physical world and to grasp its changing temperament.
42   "On Writing" first appeared in *The New York Times Book Review* as "A Storyteller's Shoptalk" (15 February 1981) and was reprinted in *Short Short Stories* (1982), ed. by J. David and J. Redfern, 199–202. Toronto: Holt, Rinehart and Winston of Canada.
43   "Creating an atmosphere" is, for example, one of the sections available on the company's internet site with the purpose of guiding the client in the choice of details that will make the difference in bringing change to their house.

To summarise and conclude, the word "atmosphere" possesses a fundamental advantage; although implanted on a complex definition, it is extremely intelligible, given its strong historical continuity. Its appeal resides in the effortless state of being identifiable that distinguishes it, in addition to its innate generosity of multiple meanings.

III
ATLAS OF ATMOSPHERES

1. *Network*

"Our perceptions and experiences of the world are significantly conditioned and altered by architecture," Juhani Pallasmaa exhorts us to consider. "A natural phenomenon, such as a storm, for instance, is a totally different condition when experienced through the device of a human construction when compared to confronting it in untamed nature" (2011a, 53). It should also be noted that "it is not possible for man to conceive a spatial vision that is not architectural; the space in which we live and move is always divided and organised architectonically" (Giberti 2012, 15). Living spaces necessarily become the preferred arena in which the human being enters into contact with atmospheres. "An occupied space creates an atmosphere," explains Niklas Luhmann (1927–1998), one of the foremost exponents of German sociology in the twentieth century. "Atmosphere is always what the individual objects that occupy places are not, the other side of their form, what perishes along with them" (2000, 112).

The impalpable nature of the atmospheric event is, as shown in the previous chapters, the guiding force that has driven the atmospheric frenzy to the point of legitimizing it. To the extent that today there are those who maintain that *architecture is nothing but atmosphere*, since "architecture [...] produces atmospheres in everything it creates" (Böhme 1991, 36). Architectural culture recognises various types of atmosphere. Such variants can be the product of ideas cultivated within the discipline or the result of borrowings derived from other fields of research.

> Atmosphere is a word that readily falls from the lips of meteorologists, on the one hand, and aestheticians, on the other. They seem, however, to mean very different things by it. [...] Aesthetics finds the atmosphere in relations among solid things — whether human or non-human, animate or inanimate. Meteorology finds it in the immaterial ether that surrounds them. (Ingold 2012, 75; 81)

The anthropologist Tim Ingold, for years an important point of reference in atmospheric investigation, above all from a socio-ecological perspective,[1] sought an integrative formula that could combine and mediate the two concepts, humanist and scientific respectively, which at first sight would appear to exclude each other (2012). He detects a possible interpretative answer in the perceptive-affective reading of the world; and doing so takes up the theories on *smooth space* put forward by Gilles Deleuze and Félix Guattari (1987), as well as some of the later writings of Maurice Merleau-Ponty (1964, 1968).

Following the example of Professor Ingold, and his conciliatory approach to the relations between antithetic principles, I sounded out the terrain in which architectural knowledge has dispersed the atmospheric seed over the course of the years. Moving between two borders of contrasting meaning, I studied every form of intelligible declination and plotted them on a map. The result was a rhizomatic map that expands and contracts at its nodal points, differentiating a chain of extremely articulated *atmospheric typicality*. Every node in the network hinges on the indissoluble and unique connection being set up, on different levels (for example, sensorial, perceptual, mental, and symbolic), between the subject and their architectonic surroundings. Emerging from this reconnaissance trip was a taxonomy that is intentionally inexact, and lacking in clear watersheds. A layering of gradual steps was generated, that is never stable and that, in thrashing out the theme of atmosphere, contemplates it — mainly — under three profiles: as a *physical element*, as a *means of socio-cultural signification*, and as a *spatial correlate of the personal experience*. There is no hierarchy among these recognised meanings, much less route rules within the mesh of the map. To plan a necessary first course of research, I took on a suggestion from the philosopher Peter Sloterdijk, respected cartographer of the atmospheric reality.[2]

> It [...] seems most prudent for theory to follow the most expanded form of atmospheric description in science, namely meteorology and climatology, in a first phase of self-assurance before devoting itself to more culturally and humanly relevant air and climate phenomena in a second step. (Sloterdijk 2016, 158)

---

1   Tim Ingold's principal contributions on the atmospheric theme can be found in the following texts: Ingold 2011, 2012, 2015, 2016.
2   See Sloterdijk 2009, 2011, 2014, 2016.

Therefore, I have chosen to start the analysis from the organisation of architectural atmosphere as a material category, to then let it branch off to more abstract and subjective horizons. The pattern of reasoning, I stress, should not be read as a fixed and unidirectional vector, but rather as a web of allusions. It consists of a subtle but powerful interconnected whole, a coherent and centrifugal system, in which the *physical pole* (atmosphere as a gassy shell) and the *spiritual pole* (atmosphere as an inner space) take on a diametrically opposite position, but not necessarily pre-eminent in importance, with respect to the centrality of the relationship between individual and architectonic work. The map is based on a non-linear geometry, assembled on a framework of concentric circles, on which connections are superimposed like the spokes of a wheel, creating semantic islands that are autonomous but fluidly tied to their neighbours. From here we have the impression that atmosphere is never fully a single experience, but a reciprocal pressure of similar experiences.

2. *Nodes*

Inside the architectural enclosure of atmospheres, the first — essential — distinction is on one side the technological-applied concreteness of the *climate control*,[3] on the other the figurative allusion to the sphere of *personal feeling*.[4] Between these two opposite poles an ample network of expressive versions is articulated, inside which some nodes appear firmer and more recurrent than others — some more comprehensive, others merely sketched. It is discontinued and variable progress that witnesses the fullness of the subject treated, the shapeless mass of which we have only scratched the surface to bring order. The entries in this map are, in the final analysis, those with which one could synthesize the architecture domain overall.

First node: atmosphere as microclimate

Atmosphere is contemplated as the ensemble of the air's thermal, hygrometric, and physicochemical factors that characterise a closed, climate-controlled space, which is to say, removed from the direct action of meteorological events (such as rain, wind, and snow). This is the most

---

3   Physical pole: atmosphere as a microclimatic bubble, which can influence the psychophysical comfort of the individual.
4   Spiritual pole: atmosphere as *Stimmung*, a state of mind, radiated with the architectonic scenario.

material dimension that atmospheric practice experiences in the architectural field, that which is literally tied to natural phenomena and, as a consequence, to the measurable variables associated with it and the general laws that govern it. Humankind has learned to modify these energies to their own advantage, at any level: from the comfortable atmosphere of "a simple cross-ventilated living room," optimised thanks to "its specific pattern of air currents, which is normally perceived by our senses of temperature and of touch" (Neutra 1954, 148), to the unpredictable effects of *geoengineering* (or *climate engineering*), in other words of the techniques of manipulation on a large scale of environmental systems that have the purpose of containing the impact of climate change.[5] The sciences of atmospheric control (of micro and macro approach) are based on a specific substantial preparatory literature, are monitored in designated government programmes, and are inserted in university courses, some of which are highly innovative. Under this accepted meaning (atmosphere as microclimate), every aspect of the atmospheric process is deciphered with the greatest rigour.

When we speak of atmosphere as microclimate, we are referring above all to the attention given to managing the interior atmosphere, charged with making buildings work. There was a time, not so long ago, that men spent most of their existence out in the open. Modern human beings have basically become "an indoor species" (Bessoudo 2017, 77). Today, the life constructed in the West (or, more generally, in the industrialised world) is spent inside closed rooms, bubbles (fixed or mobile) whose external shell and efficient technology ensure the production of a synthetic, anaesthetised environment sophisticatedly fashioned to the physiological needs of the user. Twenty-first century society is dominated by *in vitro* experiences, which is to say by experiences that are incubated and used up in man-made spaces. These boxed in spaces, in which people live, conjure up the image of the provocative "plastic bubble dome," described by Reyner Banham; namely: the inflatable polythene terephthalate shell (*environment-bubble*), which the British critic conceptualized in the mid-sixties as a design-manifesto with which to respond to "the mechanical invasion" (1965, 70) spreading through the construction sector at the time.

---

5   This is a sort of plan b, rejected by the scientific community until a few years ago because it was considered dangerously Promethean. For example, in the attempt to combat the effects of global warming, geoengineering hypothesizes an injection of chemical substances and reflective micro-particles into the stratosphere to repel some solar radiation and cool the planet.

The car, in short, is already doing quite a lot of the standard-of-living package's job — the smoochy couple dancing to the music of the radio in their parked convertible have created a ballroom in the wilderness [...] and all this is paradisal till it starts to rain. Even then, you're not licked — it takes very little air pressure to inflate a transparent Mylar airdome, the conditioned-air output of your mobile package might be able to do it, with or without a little boosting, and the dome itself, folded into a parachute pack, might be part of the package. [...] The basic proposition is simply that the power-membrane should blow down a curtain of warmed/cooled/conditioned air around the perimeter of the windward side of the un-house, and leave the surrounding weather to waft it through the living space [...]. The distribution of the air-curtain will be governed by various electronic light and weather sensors, and by that radical new invention, the weathervane. (Banham 1965, 76)

The concept of well-tempered environment theorized by Reyner Banham (1969) has materialised over time in the creation of hermetically sealed domestic and work spaces, in which the interior atmosphere is artificially manipulated and made to conform to severe standards of *well-being*, fixed at an international level.[6] Banham, assimilating the technological utopias of those years (above all the messages of Archigram), hails the construction of universalized microclimates capable of shattering any relationship with the outside: "for anyone who is prepared to foot the consequent bill for power consumed, it is now possible to live in almost any type or form of house one likes to name in any region of the world that takes the fancy." Exogenous conditions no longer represent a limit for survival: "given this convenient climatic package one may live under low ceilings in the humid tropics, behind thin walls in the arctic and under uninsulated roofs in the desert" (Banham 1969, 187). Before him, Le Corbusier had the same convictions. They are expressed in the passage with which he concludes the conference entitled *Techniques are the Very Basis of Poetry — They Open a New Cycle in Architecture*, Saturday 5 October 1929, in Buenos Aires.

What is the basis of life? *Breathing*.
Breathing what? Hot, cold, dry, damp?
Breathing pure air at a constant temperature and a regular degree of humidity.
[...] The Russian house, the Parisian, at Suez or in Buenos Aires, the luxury liner crossing the Equator will be hermetically sealed. In winter it is warm

---

6   Think, for example, of the national thermal limits in force, descended from common European directives. The range of temperatures imposed is that considered optimal for daily living and working. They were calculated by international experts who study the so-called "climate comfort" as well as by the World Health Organization.

inside, in summer cool, which means that at all times there is *clean air* inside at *exactly* 18°. The house is sealed fast! No dust can enter it. Neither flies nor mosquitos. No noise! (Le Corbusier 2015, 64–66: original italics)

Today, this orthodox faith in progress, in the imperturbable withdrawal from any kind of communication with the outside and surrounding conditions, has faded: we are aware that it is necessary, if nothing else in terms of ecological redress, to find a balance, or rather a sustainable compromise between living needs and the available resources. The same applies with regard to atmospheric climate control: "humans create their own climate; not according to free choice, however, but under preexisting, given and handed-down conditions" (Sloterdijk 2011, 46–48). Protected in air-conditioned spheres, fruit of meticulous atmospheric calculations, contemporary man, seduced and spoiled by modern comforts, has become accustomed to the high-tech reproduction of their habitat: a bubble of wellness (both physical and psychological), that encloses a fictitious, domesticated, welcoming nature, able to satisfy the user's requests and further hone their psychosomatic sensibility.

Numerous architects in the current day explore the microclimatic domain of architectural atmospheres, converting technological demands into the bases for critical-theoretical reasoning. Among them are the previously mentioned Philippe Rahm[7] and Studio AS+,[8] established by Iñaki Ábalos and Renata Sentkiewicz. In their case, thermodynamic principles become insights not so much into the physical and marked boundaries of the architectonic space, as its invisible but essential forms such as air. The equilibrium of the atmospheric ecosystem is placed at the centre of the design exercise.

The aim of manipulating the atmospheric microclimate becomes increasingly polarised, out of obvious necessity, in the hypotheses of architecture directed at combating hostile surroundings — or rather extreme contexts (for the most part natural), where the native atmosphere does not suit human life, such as deserts, marine gulfs, Arctic ice, postwar scenarios, or spatial outposts. As an example, we might think of the luxury apartments built underground, intentionally arranged to cope with unexpected events such as a collapse of the world economy, a natural

---

7   Cf., within the second chapter, the subchapter entitled "Architectural Genealogy." See also, Décosterd and Rahm 2002; Rahm 2009, 2015.
8   See Ábalos and Sentkiewicz 2015.

calamity, or a nuclear disaster.[9] A monolithic dome in concrete covers the site, defending it: the structure, resistant to over eight hundred kilometres per hour winds, transforms into a gadget that produces and gathers purified atmospheric fluid, to assist vital processes. The reference to the geodetic domes by Richard Buckminster Fuller (1895–1983) is immediate: one principally recalls the City Dome, the giant dome over the centre of Manhattan, in New York City, that he designed in 1968 with Shoji Sadao (Hays 2008). It was intended to preserve the urban organism from various types of pollution, among which acoustic pollution produced by aircrafts: "we will soon have to rename our planet 'Poluto'" (77), foretold Fuller in 1969. His project aims at the improvement of the global urban atmosphere as well as the retention of enough energy to control the climate within the whole metropolitan area. The cover Fuller proposed measured two miles in diameter and a mile and half in height. Inside it doesn't rain or snow, and the temperature is artificially regulated. It appears to be a version — more architectonic, so more material, more solid — of today's geoengineering theories, anticipating their aims. In conclusion, with Bucky Fuller's utopian domes we witness the plastic expansion of the atmospheric element from microclimatic bubble to macroclimatic infrastructure.

Second node: atmosphere as meteorological staging

Atmosphere can be interpreted and lived as a design gesture, which works with phenomena of terrestrial atmosphere and their variations. Meteorological phenomena, daily observable in nature, can be grouped into three main categories: those that concern processes tied to the distribution of heat (through, for example, wind, breezes, and draughts); those due to

---

9 A highly publicised case is the Survival Condo Project complex (www.survivalcondo.com). Designed to house up to seventy-five people for an uninterrupted time frame of up to five years, it was dug into the Atlas F missile silo, built by the Army Corps of Engineers in the seventies in Kansas, near Wichita. To recreate an authentic terrestrial atmosphere (not least to reduce the risk of residents suffering attacks of depression), special LED windows were inserted in the reinforced concrete walls. The windows, looking out on an inexistent exterior were programmed to replicate "natural" variable levels of light, changing at dawn and dusk, and able to simulate any panorama. For example, a potential client, resident in New York City, wanted a video of Central Park: "all four seasons, day and night. [...] She wanted the sounds, the taxis and the honking horns." See Osnos, Evan. 2017. "Survival of the Richest: Why Some of America's Wealthiest People are Prepping for Disaster." *The New Yorker* (print edition), 30 January 2017: 36–45.

processes involved in the water cycle (both of radiative origin, such as steam and clouds, and of perturbative character, such as rainfall and tornadoes); and finally, those generated by processes linked to atmospheric electricity (such as lightning). Essentially, there are three physical quantities in play: temperature, pressure, and humidity; adjusting, settling, and altering their balance produce different meteorological scenarios, such as rain, fog, wind, and so on. A fourth entity is generally present with these: light.

If manipulated with sensuality, understood as the capacity to artistically reproduce the impression of reality picked up by the senses, architecture can assume the consistency of air. It transforms into swarms of smoke and mist. It dematerializes. But it is there — dissolved in a delicate setting in dialogue with our body, which becomes the threshold of multiple perceptions.[10] "Air envelopes us in sensual effect," states Malte Wagenfeld. "It can warm or chill us, it carries smell and sound; breezes stimulate the skin, and wind can literally move us; sometimes we can even taste the air" (2015b, 118). In the course of studying the atmospheres of interior environments, the Australian researcher focuses on that empty space, range of the air's existence, which in architectural practice offers many design opportunities. Wagenfeld identified and catalogued a series of key phenomena that, if arranged among themselves, contribute to setting the atmospheric experience, which he conceives as multisensorial excitement, stimulated by different components and properties of the air — aesthetic medium par excellence. In this way, the project *Catalogue of Atmospheric Phenomena* (2013) came to life. Although not yet either complete or definitive, the author hopes it may function as "a perceptual model and a conceptual toolbox with which to envision atmosphere as a design

---

10   An example of this metamorphosis of the architectonic body in air sculpture is offered by the installation *Cloudscape*, designed by the Japanese studio Tetsuo Kondo Architects in collaboration with Transsolar, a climate engineering firm. The work was shown at the 12th International Architecture Exhibition in Venice (entitled *People Meet in Architecture* and directed by Kazuyo Sejima): 29 August — 21 November 2010. See Sejima, Kazuyo (ed.). 2010. *People Meet in Architecture*. Venezia: Marsilio. Without a doubt, the principle of atmospheric poetics that substantiate *Cloudscape* owes a debt to the project with which the American studio Diller Scofidio + Renfro thrilled visitors to the Swiss expo in 2002: the *Blur Building* was a temporary pavilion created on Lake Neuchâtel at Yverdon-les-Bains, in which the metallic structure disappeared in a cloud of steam. See Fernández-Galiano, Luis (ed.). 2020. *AV Monografías / Monographs* 221 (Diller Scofidio + Renfro, 2000–2020): 10–13.

typology" (2015a, 14). It is an abacus that interprets the aeriform substance in twenty formulas for use.

Air becomes the material that is shaped in order to stage an atmospheric epiphany. However, to be perceived it needs to be manifested, to allude to a certain corporeity as well as to establish a domain, free from obstructions, in which to spread and swirl. We find air converted into *haze*, hinting at colour and consistency, roughing out notes of movement, and inviting contact. As the British literary scholar Steven Connor notes, "haze is itself an interference phenomenon, in several senses" (2010, 192).

> First of all, its optical effects come about because of the scattering of light rays by minute droplets of water suspended in the air. But it also embodies what might be called an interference of registers, a compounding of light and matter. Haze represents the interchange between the palpable and the impalpable, light made semi-solid. [...] Haze is a pervasive, versatile image of the signifying resistance — a resistance out of which signification comes — of the atmosphere. (Connor 2010, 192)

The translation of the concept of atmosphere into meteorological staging, put forward as a performance by intangible but perceptible actors that take over the constructed matter, substituting it with the rarefied presence of bright spectres and clouds of steam, has been experimented — and still today is in a dynamic period of research — in the area of art. The theatrical potential of air is extremely fervid. A large number of contemporary artists have taken on the atmospheric dimension, creating authentic sensorial architectures, which trigger a strong emotional involvement. "Obviously, one cannot plan atmosphere, as it is co-produced by the people who employ the space, but it is possible to nurture an atmosphere, to allow it to grow."[11] So said the Danish artist of Icelandic origins Olafur Eliasson,[12] an icon of atmospheric sensitivity, both from a point of view of creative intensity and in terms of media exposure. The assortment of atmospheric works that he has made — pure architectural poetry — is noteworthy.[13]

---

11 The excerpt was taken from an interview by the artist Olafur Eliasson for the journal *Domus*, with regard to his Cirkelbroen project, a footbridge, made up of five circular platforms, inaugurated in 2015 in the port of Copenhagen. See Eliasson, Olafur. 2015. "Cirkelbroen." *Domus* (online), 25 August 2015: n.p. — www.domusweb.it, last accessed 15 May 2021.
12 Born in 1967, Olafur Eliasson is the same age as the architect Philippe Rahm.
13 See Eliasson 2016.

In particular, six episodes spring to mind: 1. — the multiform sensorial journey in *The Mediated Motion* (Bregenz, Austria: Kunsthaus, 2001) put forward an immersive walk in evocations of landscape, created through smells, fog, water, mushrooms, plants, wood, and soil; 2. and 3. — the polychrome fog rooms in *Your Atmospheric Colour Atlas* (Kanazawa, Japan: 21st Century Museum of Contemporary Art, 2009) and in *Feelings are Facts* (Beijing, China: Ullens Centre for Contemporary Art, 2010) reveal indeterminable spaces, apparently without edges, saturated with dense steam, which mixes with streaks of light coming from multicoloured fluorescent tubes; 4. — a colossal reproduction of the sun stuns the spectator in *The Weather Project* (London, England: Tate Modern, Turbine Hall, 2013), where a mixture of water and sugar simulates a blanket of fog, while a disc made of orange monochrome light-bulbs has the job of recreating the fiery sun itself; 5. — the hazy rain in *Fog Assembly* (Versailles, France: Château de Versailles, Bosquet de l'Étoile, 2016), in its ephemeral whirling, obliterates the edges of objects and visitors standing in it; 6. — the changing waterfall in *Rainbow Assembly* (Seoul, South Korea: Leeum, Samsung Museum of Art, 2016; Beijing, China: Red Brick Art Museum, 2018) is enchanting due to the delicate curtain of nebulised water, which seems to dance, in a scattering effect of light falling down from above. The atmospheric work of Olafur Eliasson is at the centre of numerous academic debates and artistic-architectural criticism.[14] His direct theoretical contribution appears to best advantage in the installations that he completes and opens to the public (profusely documented in their respective catalogues)[15] or in preparatory works;[16] although he also expresses himself in writing, sometimes in forms that are distant from canonical essays.[17]

This type of atmospheric sensibility, of which Eliasson has made himself a prominent representative, is deeply rooted in the creative imagination of architects from the countries in the North of Europe. Confirmation of this can be seen in the installation with which Greenland participated in the 16th International Architecture Exhibition in Venice. *Conditions*[18] is the name of

---

14   See Frichot 2008; Borch 2014; Pallasmaa 2017.
15   Particularly noteworthy, Eliasson 2010.
16   An example is the installation *Atmospheric Life Study* (Studio Olafur Eliasson, 2011). See Eliasson 2012.
17   See Eliasson 2018.
18   *Conditions*, an installation by Dorte Mandrup, Venice: Arsenale, 16th International Architecture Exhibition (entitled *Freespace* and directed by Yvonne Farrell and Shelley McNamara): 26 May — 25 November 2018. The title *Conditions* alludes

the performance staged by the Danish studio Dorte Mandrup A/S: a model to the scale of 1:12, which sketches the structure of the imminent Icefjord Centre,[19] is shown in a sensorial storm that lasts six minutes. Visitors are invited to go into a completely white, empty room, with curvilinear surfaces whose corners are softened, illusorily suspended in time and space. In front of the visitor, mute and inert, is a geometric ridge, formed by a chain of bright white triangles. At the ends of the chain the triangles have a regular shape. As we gradually move to the centre, the chain begins to twist on itself, distorting the pure figure of the polygons; the closer they are to the centre the more they are subjugated to the tension. All of a sudden, the milky, silent stillness that reigns in the room is broken: the sublime and glacial burst in. Due to the play of lights, sounds, and air movements, the natural atmosphere of those fragile and extreme lands is evoked: freezing winds blow, the space is imbued with tenuous colours recreating the flicker of the aurora borealis, and steam emerges from the floor as if the ice were burning. The architecture staged is not recounted through its consistency, its size, or the details of its construction; it is the pervading atmosphere that results the best contrivance to achieve that particular spatial experience. The intention is explained by the designer:[20] "our ambition has been to create a sensuous installation [...], which expresses the extreme natural conditions which have defined the building — more than a mere presentation of the building itself."

The dematerialization process of the architectural action does not necessarily lead to the claim of universality, displacement, and abstraction of the given context. Many installations, although working with crude substances and ancestral sensorial instincts, are *site-specific*, that is, expressly elaborated to conform to the characteristics of the place accommodating them. Or again, the process of dematerialization of the architectural action can, by paradox, lead to a physical recomposition of the intangible properties of the environment that generated it. Which

---

to the challenges deriving from the extreme climatic conditions of the site. See the two-volume catalogue dedicated to the Architecture Biennale 2018: Farrell, Yvonne, and McNamara, Shelley (eds.). 2018. *Freespace*. Venezia: La Biennale di Venezia.
19 The Icefjord Centre is the new visitor centre planned for the west coast of Greenland, near the village of Ilulissat and the old glacier Sermeq Kujalleq, a UNESCO heritage site, about three hundred kilometres above the Arctic Circle.
20 The explanation provided by Dorte Mandrup was taken from an article published online, on the site of Studio Dorte Mandrup A/S: "Taking Freespace to an Arctic Extreme." 22 May 2018, n.p. — www.dortemandrup.dk, last accessed 15 May 2021.

is to say: the structure is broken down into a group of abstract values, with which the atmospheric identity is synthesized, to then re-design the latter through corporeal manifestations, which make it perceptible. The metaphor of air, and more generally of the other atmospheric elements, also returns in this case. However, it is translated into physical structures. An example might help clarify the last two points: Venice, 57th International Art Exhibition, Israeli Pavilion.[21] The artist Gal Weinstein's project, despite being extremely complex due to its implicit allusions to the concept of time and the collective history of his people, is interesting in this situation, for the use he makes of unusual materials for artistic-architectural purposes — such as mould, rust, coffee grains, and sugared water. These become the ingredients to create sensorial sculptures alluding to architectonic masses that are not there: the imposing blackened cloud in dusty, rusty acrylic fibre originates from the same presuppositions of inquiry into the atmospheric resource that guide Olafur Eliasson's meteorological analysis. In essence, there are two parameters and terms of judgment that change: the presence of air is no longer only hinted at, but assumes a visible and ponderous consistency; the atmosphere is seen to reflect negative tonalities too, apparent in the mind-numbing smell of mildew that saturates the entire space.

The examples taken from the world of contemporary art and relative descriptions, whose aim was to reproduce the emotional impact of single orchestrated experiences, are a further invitation to respond — on a design level — to the call of atmosphere's potential. "Once again," as Harry Francis Mallgrave points out, talking in specific about the ability of light to organise atmospheric meanings, "contemporary art and its inter-disciplinary collaborations offer an instructive example of how 'atmosphere' might be more seriously considered" (2013, 159). An intermediary step, established to contribute to a more informed assimilation of what atmosphere can bring to the evolution of architectural design, can be identified in the effort to mediate the artistic message that architecture cultivates within itself and that is a horizon of infinite possibilities. As Juhani Pallasmaa explains, the

---

21 *Sun Stand Still*, exhibition curated by Tami Katz-Freiman hosting a site-specific installation by Gal Weinstein, Venice: Giardini della Biennale, 57th International Art Exhibition (entitled *Viva Arte Viva* and directed by Christine Macel): 13 May — 26 November 2017. See the two-volume catalogue dedicated to the Art Biennale 2017: Macel, Christine (ed.). 2017. *Viva Arte Viva*. New York: Rizzoli International Publications.

artistic value of an architectural experience resides in its capacity to evoke and amplify emotions.

A powerful experience of architecture likewise turns our attention outside itself. The artistic value of great architectural works is not in their material existence or aesthetic essence but the images and emotions that they evoke in the observer. A great building makes us experience gravity, time and — ultimately — ourselves, in a strengthened and meaningful way. (Pallasmaa 2012b, 173)

Third node: atmosphere as aesthetic-decorative quality

Atmospheric effect is sought after in the epidermal cladding of the architectonic object or, more precisely, in its decorative apparatus, made up of visible components, such as the colour, texture, and materiality of the surfaces — irrespective of the ambient conditions in the surroundings. There is, therefore, a shift in paradigm with respect to the two previous points: atmospheric power no longer adopts the aeriform substance, either to domesticate it to the psychophysical needs of the users or to direct it in a choreography of meteorological events, it projects onto the skin of the architectonic body, which becomes a substrate fertile with atmospheric impressions. Atmosphere abandons the empty space and settles on a rigid support, that is for the most part two-dimensional, solid but not fully immersive.

Listed among the authors who have contributed an aesthetic-decorative interpretation to the atmospheric process is Gottfried Semper (Wigley 1998a). He maintains that the factors determining the formation of an atmosphere should be traced to the decorative backdrop that wraps the faces of a building like a garment. Anastasia Karandinou noted that for Semper (1803–1879) "the essence of a space is correlated to the effect of the things' physical surface, and is regarded as independent from the density of the in-between space" (2013, 18). The shell, conceived as a shield, masks the structural framework and the ensemble of construction elements, letting the structure serve as support on which to hoist the exterior arrangement of symbols, signs, and suggestions. A few decades later, Louis Henry Sullivan (1856–1924) recognises that bare buildings, if "clad in a garment of poetic imagery, half hid as it were in choice products of loom and mine, [appeal] with redoubled power" ([1892] 1979, 187). Which would be true, since a building knowingly decorated, "that is to say, a building which is truly a work of art," "is in its nature, essence and physical being an emotional expression" (Sullivan, 188). Hence the architectonic shell, in this case too, as for Gottfried Semper, becomes the threshold steeped in atmospheric tension: the emotional impulses flow harmoniously throughout its parts, occurring in greater depth in "mass-composition" but with greater intensity in "decorative ornamentation" (Sullivan, 188).

The main factor to shape the emotional expressiveness of architectonic cladding (expressiveness intelligible both on perceptual and symbolic levels) is the reactivity of the materials. They are revealed to be an efficient expedient to influence the way in which an individual experiences a space. A latent potential is rooted in materials that — if appropriately prompted — is able to activate the unique characteristics of any substance, even the most conventional, converting it into an opportunity for atmospheric priming, that is of contact (not necessarily physical) between the surfaces and the observer. Each material, writes Juhani Pallasmaa, conveys its atmospheric identity, reflecting its own specific story.

> Materials and surfaces have languages of their own. Stone speaks of its distant geological origins, its durability and inherent permanence. Brick makes one think of earth and fire, gravity, and the ageless traditions of construction. Bronze evokes the extreme heat of its manufacture, the ancient processes of casting, and the passage of time as measured by its patina. Wood speaks of its two existences and time scales; its first life as a growing tree and the second as a human artefact made by the caring hand of the carpenter or cabinetmaker. (Pallasmaa 2016a, 177–178)

Materials give life to artistic and architectonic works that "awaken bodily experiences of weight and gravity" and that, as a consequence, "directly address our skeletal and muscular system" (Pallasmaa 2000, 80) in the moment in which we observe them. This reading of atmospheric surfaces as emotionally resonant places recalls the analysis of the French philosophers Gilles Deleuze and Félix Guattari with respect to facial expressiveness, in other words its ability to elicit reactions in others. "The face is not an envelope exterior to the person who speaks, thinks, or feels" (1987, 167). On the contrary, "the face constructs the wall that the signifier needs in order to bounce off of; it constitutes the wall of the signifier, the frame or screen" (Deleuze and Guattari, 168). On a par with a wall, "the face is a surface: facial traits, lines, wrinkles; long face, square face, triangular face; the face is a map" (170).

The materiality of architecture is made up as much of visible as invisible elements, which convert cladding into communicative interfaces that can establish a perceptual link with whoever explores it with attention, or simply brushes against it. Even before being attentively observed, clarifies Juhani Pallasmaa, materials can provide multiple sensorial impressions about their qualities thanks to the messages gathered from the action of touching.

> We are not usually aware that an unconscious experience of touch is unavoidably concealed in vision. As we look, the eye touches, and before we even see an object, we have already touched it and judged its weight, temperature and surface texture. [...] Touch is the unconsciousness of vision, and this hidden tactile experience determines the sensuous qualities of the perceived object. (Pallasmaa 2009a, 101–102)

A material can produce different effects according to how it is employed and treated; the decorative stamp influencing its aspect plays a fundamental role in the generation of tactile simulations, emotional resonance, and affective evocations. In conclusion, "the charm of materials [...] lies largely in their atmospheric potentiality" (Griffero 2014a, 97).

Contemporary architecture is witnessing an intensification in the atmospheric expressivity of its surfaces, overwhelmed by the phenomenon of architecture as performance (Canepa 2018). Creative and economic efforts are focused on the shape of the building, insisting on the extravagance of volumes, the cult of facadism, and the glorification of the shell. In particular, concentration on the exterior cladding (the so-called "skin") has matured into a veritable obsession; experiments on materials, textures, patterns, graphics, transparencies, and colours abound. Green, multimedia, robotised, high performance: the shell-surfaces of buildings are given the importance of manifestoes with which designers affirm their identity and authoritativeness. To the extent that today architects seem to be more interested in the atmospheres produced by the exterior aspects of their buildings than those inspired by the inner spatiality, whose design is often delegated to other professionals, such as interior designers, or in any case to third parties (Moussavi and Kubo 2008). The aesthetic-decorative charge that makes these atmospheric facades vibrate — almost as though they were theatrical backdrops — reverberate around their surroundings, forming the atmospheric charisma of the urban organism in its entirety.

Fourth node: atmosphere as the identity of a place

Atmosphere is the echo of the *genius loci*, the Latin locution commonly translated as "character of a place." Just like the notion of atmosphere, the *genius loci* is a vague, abstract concept largely employed in the metaphorical sense if not actually rhetorically; the term has an ancient history, burying its roots in the classical idea of the sacredness of places, present in both Greek and Latin culture. The risk, as Tonino Griffero notes (2015), is that we are too quick to say that a place possesses a *genius locus*, in other words a patrimony of unique and inimitable characteristics, which guarantee the identity and authenticity of whoever lives there. "The argument adopted in favour of place-identity is," indeed, "usually the cliché that the *genius loci* is the *quid* that transforms an anonymous space into an intensely expressive lived place" (Griffero 2020a, 138).

In view of, or because of its inherent ambiguity, the expression *genius loci* suffers an arduous state of inflation due to the use made of it in different disciplines, each of which assimilates and changes its form to meet its aims and tools. In the architectural field, two authors explicitly interested in the theme were Aldo Rossi ([1966] 1984) and Christian Norberg-Schulz (1979). The Italian architect Aldo Rossi (1931–1997) introduces the concept of *locus*.

> The *locus* is a relationship between a certain specific location and the buildings that are in it. It is at once singular and universal. [...] Perhaps we can better understand the concept of *locus*, which at times seems rather opaque, by approaching it from another perspective, by penetrating it in a more familiar, more visible — even if no longer rational — way. Otherwise, we continue to grasp at outlines which only evaporate and disappear. These outlines [...] trace the relation of architecture to its location — the place of art — and thereby its connections to, and the precise articulation of, the *locus* itself as a singular artifact determined by its space and time, by its topographical dimensions and its form, by its being the seat of a succession of ancient and recent events, by its memory. (Rossi 1984, 103; 107)

The Norwegian architect Christian Norberg-Schulz (1926–2000) dedicates an entire book to the principle of the *genius loci*, to give structure to years of research. In *Genius Loci: Towards a Phenomenology of Architecture*, he writes that "architecture means to visualize the *genius loci*" (1979, 5), namely "the 'spirit of place' which the ancients recognized as that 'opposite' man has to come to terms with, to be able to dwell" (10–

11). Norberg-Schulz's position is particularly interesting in the passage where he clarifies the atmospheric basis.

> The structure of place ought to be [...] analyzed by means of the categories "space" and "character." Whereas "space" denotes the three-dimensional organization of the elements which make up a place, "character" denotes the general "atmosphere" which is the most comprehensive property of any place. [...] "Character" is at the same time a more general and a more concrete concept than "space." On the one hand it denotes a general comprehensive atmosphere, and on the other the concrete form and substance of the space-defining elements. Any real *presence* is intimately linked with a character. [...] In general we have to emphasize that *all places have character*, and that character is the basic mode in which the world is "given." (Norberg-Schulz 1979, 11; 13–14: original italics)

Today, many of the more prominent names in the research into the atmospheric phenomenon combine the concept of *genius loci* with that of atmosphere. For Juhani Pallasmaa, the spirit of the place is a feature of the human experience that is so ephemeral, confusedly blurred, and immaterial that it is instinctive to closely correlate it to atmosphere. On which note, Pallasmaa speaks of "the atmosphere of a place" (2014a, 231), an expression that recognises and confers to a place the identity that distinguishes it as well as circumscribing its inborn perceptual specificity, capable of standing out despite the variety of its constituent parts. Tonino Griffero promotes the idea of studying the construct of the *genius loci*, which currently drives the debate in philosophy and humanities chiefly in a metaphorical sense, through an "atmospheric approach" (2015): with this in mind, "a place has its own *genius* only if (when and where) it radiates an intense and authoritative specific atmosphere" (Griffero 2020a, 146). Harry Francis Mallgrave enters into his personal treatment of architectural atmospheres (2018, chapter VII), lingering on the dichotomy between "space" and "place": this last emerging as "the humanization or enculturation of space" (Mallgrave, 118). In a brief historical excursus (in which he cites, among others, Bruno Zevi, Rudolf Schwartz, and Kevin Lynch), Mallgrave configures his reasoning setting out from the dual notions of *existential space* and *architectural space*,[22] which he reckons germinal argumentations on the essential and founding character of a given context.

---

22 Disseminated in the early seventies by Christian Norberg-Schulz (1971).

In line with this overview of theoretical positions, it is possible to hypothesize exploring an atmospheric reading of the design sensibility of some architects who have not — so far — ever been directly linked to the question of atmosphere. In doing so, it would be feasible to adopt as filters of inquiry the model of the *genius loci* and the related generating element of the *light*. As Christian Norberg-Schulz explains, "to some extent the character of a place is a function of time; it changes with the seasons, the course of the day and the weather, factors which above all determine different conditions of *light*" (1979, 14: original italics). Among the possible case studies, I would like to propose the figure of Louis Isadore Kahn (1901–1974). As will be shown, it is Kahn — the architect of geometries, mass, structure, archetypes, and universal symbolism[23] — who, through his words, puts himself forward as an architect of atmosphere.

In the volume *Idea e immagine* ("Idea and Image"), dedicated to the poetics of Louis Kahn, Christian Norberg-Schulz declares his search for an interpretive key to the concept of space fine-tuned by the great American master as well as of "his understanding the built structure as a giver of ambient character" (1980, 7). Analysing a selection of his writings and projects, he maintains that for Kahn "architecture is primarily an expression of the institutions of man, which date back to the origin in which man came to realise his 'desires' or his 'inspirations'" (Norberg-Schulz, 10). There follows the main objective of designing "a space aware of what it wants to be": "when a space is aware of what it wants to be, it becomes a *room*, or rather a place with a particular *character*" (12: original italics). "The room," confirms Louis Kahn, "is the beginning of architecture. It is the place of the mind. You in the room with its dimensions, its structure, its light respond to its character, its spiritual aura" (1973 as reprinted in 1991, 263). It doesn't matter how big or complex the space available is: even the landing of a flight of stairs could be a room. In the same way "the bay window can be the private room within a room" (265).

This montage of reflections shows the interest Louis Kahn held for the atmospheric dimension, understood as the intimate and intrinsic character of a place, on which to build — as part of a ritual — the relationships of spatiality that codify a "room," or an architectonic domain consciously planned for human activity. The formation of character precedes the planning of the intended use and anticipates the necessity for functionalization.

---

23 See Lobell 1979; McCarter 2005; Kries, Eisenbrand, and von Moos 2013.

Hence there is a strong and immediate reference to the definition of *genius loci* formalised by Christian Norberg-Schulz a few years later:[24] "the structure of a place, or the dimension where life *takes place*, is the *genius loci*. [...] The *genius* corresponds to what a thing is or to what it 'would be'" (1980, 28: original italics).

For Louis Kahn, the founding element of the character of a place is the contribution of light, or more precisely *natural light*. Light that changes from place to place, engendered by the specific nature of the site, combed by the reverberation of seasons and the passing of the hours: never the same, from instant to instant. This is the element the project hangs on, which would otherwise produce a "ridiculous building" (Kahn 1961, 10), a stereotypical identity, estranged from and disconnected to its surroundings. Light bathing a room increases its atmosphere: "light is material life. The mountains, the streams, the atmosphere is spent light" (Kahn 1973 as reprinted in 1991, 268). And from atmosphere light evolves in architecture, governed by its physical structure, however intangible it may be. "Structure is the maker of light. When you decide on the structure, you're deciding on light," declares Kahn. "In the old buildings, the columns were an expression of light, no light, light, no light, light, no light, light" (1969 as reprinted in 1991, 245). Summing itself up in the essence of light, the atmosphere of a room can be traced back to its natural roots, achieving a corporeity that from an ambient restriction becomes a design input.

> One of the things which impressed me very much during my stay in Luanda was the marked glare in the atmosphere... when you were on the interior of any building, looking at a window was unbearable because of the glare. The dark walls framing the brilliant light outside made you very uncomfortable. The tendency was to look away from the window. [...] And I thought wouldn't it be good if one could express... find an architectural expression for the problems of glare without adding devices to a window... but rather by developing a warm architecture... which somehow tells the story of the problems of glare. (Kahn 1961, 9)

A subject that is very close to that of the *genius loci* is represented by *topophilia*, the neologism that delineates the emotional tie created between

---

24 The writings and speeches of Louis Kahn examined here date to a time spanning from the early sixties to the early seventies; Christian Norberg-Schulz published the book *Genius Loci* in 1979.

human beings and their places.²⁵ According to the French philosopher Gaston Bachelard (1884–1962), the experience of topophilia attempts to determine "the human value of the sorts of space that may be grasped, [...] the space we love" (1994, XXXV). The term acquires prominence within perception studies in geography and so-called humanistic geography: for the humanistic angle, place, although also described by physical and objective data, is first and foremost subjective, experienced and perceived reality. It is in such a context that the sensibility of *genius loci* assumes importance. In particular, it is the theories of Chinese-American geographer, Professor Yi-Fu Tuan, among the leading exponents of the humanistic perspective, that develop the concept of topophilia (1974). To nurture spatial knowledge, Tuan stresses the primacy of experience, which implies the establishment of a visceral relationship with place and a rooted sense of belonging; at the same time, Tuan attributes to the context the necessity for a certain detachment from the individual, an autonomy of meaning that is honed in that "general comprehensive atmosphere" (Norberg-Schulz 1979, 13–14), *a priori* constituent of its *genius loci*.

To explain what is perceived in one's surroundings, providing precise details that can capture its every nuance, is not a simple undertaking. For Tuan (1974, chapter V) literary activity, thanks to its malleable and expressive linguistic means, proves to be an efficient expedient of communication, and certainly more incisive than the solutions provided by the social sciences. So, the spirit of the place, or the specific and intimate atmosphere of a given place, relives in topobiographical descriptions,²⁶ constructed from the image that the place offers of itself; apparently vague and picturesque, these types of description filter the overall atmospheric tone — in a subtle and involving manner.²⁷ In the fragment that follows, the Danish architect Steen Eiler Rasmussen (1898–1990) immortalises the character of the city of Boston, depicting its atmospheric identity with rapid brushstrokes: breathing its air,

---

25 "Topophilia," in *Environmental Psychology: An introduction*. 2013. Ed. by L. Steg, A.E. van den Berg, and J.I.M. de Groot, 45. Chichester: Wiley — Leicester: The British Psychological Society.
26 A topobiographical testimony is made up of three elements: the place, the memory, and the narrative voice of the individual (often in the first-person but, in any case, from their subjective point of view). To recount is to try and organise experiences into a complete framework, which includes all the meanings. Such complexity is always spatially constructed. See Karjalainen 2015.
27 "Literary language has the capacity to dwell on the complexities of spatial experience" (Havik 2019, § 4).

savouring its light, and stroking its iconic architectures — tattooists of active traces on memory.

> Walking along the shore of the Charles River in Boston, Massachusetts, in the early morning, you not only *feel* that the air is cool but you imagine that you can *see* it. Old buildings in Boston seem bright and new with sharply etched cool shadows, and scintillating gleams from sailing boats in the water make your eyes blink. But if you return to the same spot in the evening, just before sunset, you find the glaring colors of the morning now saturated and warm. The Hancock Building, which had stood gray-white and sharp against the morning sky, is now gold and red. The golden dome of the State House is seen floating in the Canaletto-like atmosphere as a second sun. You *feel* the warmth of the evening sun and you *see* its warm light. (Rasmussen 1959, 221–222: original italics)

The more vague a thing is that we have experienced and wish to recount (as in the case of the atmosphere of a place), the more precise we must be in describing it and the more skilled at communicating the effects it had on us. It might seem a paradox, but it isn't. Think of how many lines of verse poets have dedicated to the moon. A possible strategy to capture the profound essence of a place is the "extension of human identity into our environment" (Bloomer and Moore 1977, 131) by means of one's lived experiences, memories, the organization of our body, and its points of reference (Havik 2019). It involves the same mechanism of self-identification at the basis of the transformation process of words into images. Words build images if they can trigger shared experiences (being already experienced, although in different forms) and sensorial perceptions (evoked by physical, concrete, and tangible qualities). In writing, for example, a description of colours and materials serves to activate the vision and help the reader to compose the visual image that the author wants to recreate in order to make the reader feel immersed and engaged. It is exactly what Steen Eiler Rasmussen does in the above passage: his experience of the atmosphere of the city of Boston takes shape through fresh air, saturated and warm colours, the mild weather of the evening, and so on.

Fifth node: atmosphere as collective imagination

Atmosphere is the announcement of the *Zeitgeist*, the cultural spirit of the time, which serves as a vehicle of the values proper to a community, among which are social, ideological, political, and sacred values. This meaning reading is clearly highlighted by Mark Wigley.

> Architectural historians work hard to produce a sense of atmosphere, describing the historical climate within which architects work. The whole Zeitgeist mentality is atmospheric. The *geist*, the spirit of a historical moment, is a kind of wind that swirls around events. Modernity is such an atmosphere. (Wigley 1998a, 25)

Every historical period is unique, and of complex and ambiguous interpretation. To be able to understand them, we need a framework large enough to embrace the compound variety of phenomena that distinguishes them. Among these phenomena are atmospheres. The economics scholar Christian Julmi (2017) observes that, when we want to explore the atmospheric element within a specific historical context, it becomes necessary to examine the social foundation to understand why given atmospheric conditions came to be consolidated. Every atmosphere can (must) be interpreted as a situation intrinsically cast by a socio-cultural milieu. There is no civilisation or epoch that has not forged its own atmospheric identity. It echoes with the values generated by the society that has brought it to life, values that find a vigorous means of resonance in the communicative power of architecture, above all constructed architecture. The historical essence is "stored in the landscapes, in cities and buildings, stored in the objects we live with" (Havik and Tielens 2013a, 63). Peter Zumthor explains, when interviewed about the nature of atmosphere, that according to him the trigger of the atmospheric dynamics can be encapsulated in the *sense of history*; which is manifested in "old factories, industrial buildings — specifically old brick factories actually: pure constructions, full of atmosphere" (Havik and Tielens, 63).

By means of the architectures and atmospheric haloes that they give off, it is possible to perceive and decipher the prevalent ideological climate in a particular phase of history. In his essay *The Atmosphere of Moscow* (1930), Le Corbusier speaks of "the spirit of the times" as follows.

> A striking flood of plans: plans of factories, of dams, of mills, of dwellings, of entire cities. All of them under one sign: whatever brings progress. Architecture swells, moves, bestirs itself, and gives birth, breathed on and fertilized by those who know something, and those who make believe they do. [...] In addition, for the big Ford automobile factory, an American architect specializing in industrial towns was called in; what he designed looks like a prison; it is nevertheless the model American company town. But the spirit of the times is

not there; it seems anachronistic. Moscow laughs at it; it doesn't suit this new environment. This little incident is a touchstone; it gives the measure of the intellectual quality of Moscow planning. (Le Corbusier 2015, 260–261)

The cyclical changing of historical seasons, as well as their inexorable renovation and reconstruction, significantly influences not only the way in which society — with its identifying cultural tendencies and ideologies — reorganises itself, but also the way in which it is perceived. The warning comes from Walter Benjamin: "during long periods of history, the mode of human sense perception changes with humanity's entire mode of existence." "The fifth century, with its great shifts of population, saw the birth of the late Roman art industry and the Vienna Genesis," he explains, "and there developed not only an art different from that of antiquity but also a new kind of perception" ([1935] 2007, 222). In short, the ways in which we enter into contact with places change and new patterns of symbols are designed to describe them. The collective imagination formulates new atmospheres, evoked to synthesize the essence of the mutation underway. The more immediate the mediation of the collective imagination to establish a unanimously understood and excepted symbolism, the more recognisable the associated atmospheric character. Atmosphere echoes the existential meaning of a given architecture, inevitably tied to a particular spatial and temporal context.

This role of atmosphere illustrates the reason that "highly technologised settings tend to leave our emotions cold and distant": "they are unable to invite and simulate our deep primal imagery" (Pallasmaa 2011b, 131); in other words, we intuit that, if contemporary works alienate us (above all in relation to historic and natural contexts), the underlying problem consists in the "weakness of the atmospheric quality" (Pallasmaa 2014a, 244). This is why a thermal power station or a prefabricated warehouse facade generally miss the process of symbolic abstraction that converts them into atmospheric images capable of communicating specific collective values — even if they were the product of a fatuous convention tainted by prejudices. In any case, the evocative power of architectural atmospheres is widely celebrated: think of the cinema, theatre, photography, figurative painting, and literature. The justification is obvious: the architectural imagination is able to recreate "the sense of context and place, as well as the culture and historical era, for the depicted scene or event" (Pallasmaa 2011b, 121).

A further interesting aspect in the interpretation of the concept of atmosphere as the imagination of a community resides in its relationship with the tendencies sought by fashion: when we stage the atmospheric character of an excerpt of the history, often also embedded in a certain place, we use an ensemble of the signs and symbols that make up its identity, as conventionally recognised. This approach is frequently found, for example, in advertising, interior architecture, and set design, where it is possible to depict "the atmosphere of the 1920s, the atmosphere of a boudoir, a barracks-like atmosphere or also the atmosphere of elegance, of petty-bourgeoisie, of decorum, of wealth, of poverty, etc." (Böhme 2013c, 24).

Sixth node: atmosphere as metaphor

Atmosphere changes in metaphor, linked to the integrative power of words and the imagination, insofar as it is a means of signification (or re-signification). The atmosphere is planned and set up as a mental backdrop, elaborated to evoke a physical presence that isn't there or to portray some of its specific qualities that transcend the domain of the concrete and material. As Juhani Pallasmaa highlights, works of architecture are intrinsically associated with metaphorical representations, that guide and organize our spatial perception.

> The task of architecture is not only to provide physical shelter, facilitate activities and stimulate sensory pleasure. In addition to being externalisations and extensions of human bodily functions, buildings are also mental extensions and projections, they are externalisations of our imagination, memory and conceptual capacities. (Pallasmaa 2011b, 119)

Architectonic artefacts become the catalyst for our existential experiences and confer on them a very precise meaning. They can touch us.

> Architecture is an art form of inherently weak impact compared with, for instance, the flood of emotions mobilized by theatrical, cinematic and musical experiences. The strength of architectural impact derives from its unavoidable presence as the perpetual unconscious pre-understanding of our existential condition. (Pallasmaa and Zambelli 2020, 112–113)

The descriptive practice of geometry and algorithms turns out to be powerless to replicate the need for explanations of the emotional impulses and effects that architecture can stimulate. As a result we turn to metaphor, in an attempt to capture the immaterial essence that animates the architectonic body. Employed as a metaphor, atmosphere becomes a *communicative device*. For instance, when we say that the architecture of

Kazuyo Sejima and Ryūe Nishizawa[28] is "rarefied" we are employing a series of derived metaphors. The adjective, which literally means "less dense" or, in the figurative sense, "refined, subtle," was legitimized and made famous by the Italian publisher Mondadori Electa, although it had been around for some time already: "SANAA has distinguished itself by its highly original approach to projects," says the promotional release at the launch of the monograph published by Electa. "The use of elementary volumes, simple geometry, translucent materials and polycarbonate casing produces a rarefied architecture that is strikingly contemporary" (Hasegawa 2005). From that moment onwards, the metaphor of rarefied abstraction was crystallised into an inborn character of the Japanese duo's design legacy, since it was found to be valid to sift its emotional content.

All architecture generates impressions that are complex, interconnected, and multisensory: we experience and portray them in a metaphorical key, condensing them in an *ideal* atmosphere. As we saw in the first chapter, it is a characteristic of atmosphere to be inherently metaphorical. In the words of Richard Neutra, with the atmospheric dimension, "a mental perspective of space values involved as well as a mere visual foreshortening" (1954, 168) enters into play. This is why paraphrasing atmosphere as a metaphor helps to define it. Many architects, conscious of the metaphorical potential of atmospheres, have adopted them within their poetics. Jean Nouvel[29] delineates his approach in these terms: "I'm no magician, but I try to create a space that isn't legible, a space that works as the mental extension of sight." He clarifies that "this seductive space, this virtual space of illusion, is based on very precise strategies, strategies that are often diversionary" (Baudrillard and Nouvel 2002, 6). He then explains what he means by "diversion": "this diversion, which reroutes our perception of phenomena from the material to the immaterial, is a concept that architecture should appropriate for itself" (Baudrillard and Nouvel, 7). Travelling down this design path, we reach the fine-tuning of expressive settings of the author's mental universe. They achieve the objective for which they were conceived, if they manage to resonate with the sensitivity of whoever experiences those spaces, that is to say if the atmospheric metaphor is intelligible — although in an arbitrary manner.

---

28 In 2010 Sejima and Nishizawa, pupils of Toyo Ito and founders of the studio SANAA, were awarded the Pritzker Architecture Prize.
29 Jean Nouvel received the Pritzker Architecture Prize in 2008.

This occurs, notes Juhani Pallasmaa, if the existential meaning of the architectural action enclosed in the metaphor is understood.

> Authentic architectural images and metaphors re-articulate the primordial and historical essences of our existential experiences, concealed and stored in our genetic constitution and unconscious. A wall that moves us today echoes the first separation of the exterior and interior worlds; a roof that touches us makes us conscious of the climate and weather outside, and the pleasurable protection from the elements; the fireplace that gives us maximum comfort and pleasure today arises from the very invention of fire and the ageless enjoyment of the safety and domesticity of tamed fire by countless generations of our ancestors. (Pallasmaa 2011b, 127)

From this perspective, atmospheres become metaphors not only of mental space but also of physically experienced space. Harry Francis Mallgrave, taking up the "physiognomic" reading of space put forward by the art historian Heinrich Wölfflin ([1886] 1994), highlights how when we, human beings, enter into contact with buildings "we often also read the built environment in allegorical or anthropomorphic terms: the urban hardscapes of an uncaring city, the fiscal transparency of the glazed bank, the relaxing 'coziness' of a room with a fireplace" (Mallgrave 2013, 138).

Even an empty space can be atmospherically suggestive, precisely because of the potential projections of presences and actions that it inspires. There is an architectonic box and a choreography of objects, but the occupier is missing: a stone silence reigns. And yet the ensemble of details, in the moment when it is scrutinized (and therefore interpreted), orchestrates an atmosphere that is nothing if not metaphor, metaphor of experiences, relationships, and movements — of existential meanings. In the following passage, the Spanish architect Fernando Espuelas illustrates this with poetry.

> The eye of the observer, penetrating the empty enclosure, converts it into a theatre home in which every object has a precise role. Just like those plays in which the characters constantly allude to someone who never appears, so it is with objects, which when looked at refer to the absent inhabitant. The seat turned slightly away from the table, an open book, a pair of glasses, and a pipe that is slowly going out are signs of suspended life in that place, the luminous aftermath of someone who is no longer there. The objects, suggesting gestures, behaviours, sometimes stories related to the absent one, seem to want to hold the observer's attention and delay the moment in which they must return to mere materiality. When they are not looked at, they lose their attribute of being a sign of life to return to the reign of natural phenomena. (Espuelas 1999, 153–154)

Seventh node: atmosphere as constitutive character

Atmosphere is adopted as character, predisposed to confer to a given place an essential aspect that connotes it, instilling particular values, for example, emotional, sentimental, social, ideological, moral, or spiritual. In short: an identity. Atmosphere's *theatrical tone* emerges; its communicative function is fully unveiled. In contrast with the previous point, however, no conceptual metaphors are elaborated, interwoven with words and rhetorical allusions to the mental threshold, aimed at translating the abstract entity of spaces that are already developed, whether full or empty. No: in this case, it is a question of metaphors established as a design act, intentionally devised to create characterised and characterising atmospheric scenarios. The metaphor materialises, taking on its physical corporeity: it becomes a *mise-en-scène*, perceptible by gradual levels. In appearance, this interpretation of atmospheric dynamism recalls the hypothesis of "atmosphere as meteorological staging." The discrepancy lies in losing the boundaries of existence imposed by the meteorological domain so that the metaphor can also draw on references of other imaginary.

"There are no recipes, of course, in planning atmospheres" (Griffero 2014c, 35). In the first instance, to outline a rough formula of atmospheric artifice, we can draft two opposing strategies. The first strategy requires the designer to limit theirself to suggesting a potential atmospheric impression to someone faced with their architectonic space, a space that must be intentionally conceived in a "more neutral" manner, with the purpose of stimulating "the hermeneutic and emotional creativity of the user" (Griffero, 37). On the contrary, the second strategy encourages seduction of the observer, to involve them in a clearly defined design narrative that sends them emotional and/or ideological messages predetermined by the author. Atmospheres, understood as characterisation, answer to this last attitude, an overtly design-led attitude. As the French sociologist Jean-Paul Thibaud says, more than being made, atmospheres are *installed*. Setting out from the premise that "to install" means "to locate in a chosen place" (a person or a thing), such a gesture becomes "action which necessarily involves a place" (2014a, 53), from which to let oneself be inspired or conditioned. The preliminary setting not only provides the frame in which to situate the sought-after atmospheric scene, but reveals itself to be a founding element for its genesis. "Installing an atmosphere therefore always means coming to terms with an existing atmosphere, and finding ways of inflecting and transforming it" (Thibaud, 55).

To give body to atmosphere, shaping a true *atmospheric work*, appropriate raw materials are needed that are more or less tangible and able to generate emotions and mental associations. These design factors help to influence the spatial experience: they are air, colours, sounds, smells, fluctuations in temperature, and so on. The preferred material to give substance to an efficient atmospheric consistency of space is, without a doubt, *light*. "The best, most temporal way of making a building that I ever heard of is by making it with light" (1975, 157) stresses the American icon of pop art Andy Warhol (1928–1987), who, in his book *The Philosophy of Andy Warhol*, dedicates an entire chapter to the theme of atmosphere — in an impetuous stream of consciousness, in which he disperses ideas about art, time, beauty, and fame. Light has always thrilled architects, to the extent of being considered "the fundamental basis of architecture" (Le Corbusier [1930] 2015, 132).

The opportunities for interpretation that light offers are infinite: from protean creative artifice, capable of communicating the latent sense of a particular situation, it evolves, for example, into a weighty means of transmission of political intent. Warhol goes on: "the Fascists did a lot of this 'light architecture'" (1975, 157). And again: "Hitler always needed buildings in a hurry to make speeches from, so his architect created these 'buildings' for him that were illusion buildings, completely constructed by lighting effects, where he defined a very big space" (Warhol, 157–158). Taking precedence over all is the megalomaniacal ceremony of the Lichtdom, literally "cathedral of light" (1970, 59), as it was renamed by its originator, Albert Speer, the regime's architect from the age of just twenty-nine. The first trial takes place in 1933 in Nuremberg, on the zeppelin airfield, at the end of the annual Nazi party congress. To house the Führer's rally, Speer is appointed to design a new grandstand in stone to substitute the former wooden one: he takes his inspiration from the Pergamon Altar, inaugurated in that period in Berlin, and produces a grandiose transposition, enlarging its dimensions so as to be able to accommodate tens of thousands of men. With the aim of amplifying the mystical effect of the long-awaited gathering, as well as to emphasize the sense of power emanating from the architectonic bulk, a hundred and thirty motorised anti-aircraft spotlights are installed. Once turned on, they cut through the darkness, sculpting the night with strong beams of white light projected upwards, visible miles away. "The feeling was of a vast room, with the beams serving as mighty pillars of infinitely high outer walls," recounts Speer. "Now and then a cloud moved through this wreath of lights, bringing an element of surrealistic surprise to the mirage" (1970, 59).

Albert Speer's monument proves to be pure art of spatial prestidigitation, where the overall spectacular installation is attributed to an impalpable atmosphere, which acquires a symbolic solidity, strong enough to become crystallized in history. The light, an intangible substance par excellence, is not only seen, but — in the atmospheric contact — also lived, being an integral part of the architectural experience. "Light in architecture can scarcely be considered as an element itself," Harry Francis Mallgrave underlines. "In addition to its conditioning of the material qualities of the environment, it also structures the atmospheric sense of embeddedness or how one peripherally experiences a spatial environment" (2013, 159).

The atmospheric charge — due to the fascination it holds as a demiurgic force, expert in moulding the character of a space, and consequently, in influencing the way in which people feel and perceive the space — holds sway over all the contexts that originate from the start as scenery, make-believe, or spectacle. Theme parks come to mind: above all the world of Walt Disney. "Whoever returns [...] does it to re-explore that artificial but gratifying atmosphere that finds its synthesis in the sense of control, of familiarity, and necessity to dream" (Buiatti 2014, 45). Every architectural detail is designed to collaborate in the general atmospheric mise-en-scène, a unification of symbolic and sensory accents, which become relational contrivance, where environment and visitors can establish a reciprocal connection. Such a connection is not of a merely visual nature, it promotes an integral spatial involvement. According to Gernot Böhme, it is with the postmodern movement and its aesthetics of rehabilitation — also ironic and uninhibited — of the formal metaphor that awakens a new interest in the articulation of space, on the basis of the corporeal sensations felt by whoever benefits from the building.

> Seen from the theory of atmospheres architecture is not a visual art. [...] In the traditional view yes, but since postmodernity another idea of architecture is growing, the idea that the main task of architecture is not the production of sight but of space. That is to say spaces and location with a certain mood, i.e. atmospheres. (Böhme 2014, 11)

Research and the requirement for atmospherically qualified environments, capable of ensuring a marked typicality, so mesmerising one could be lost inside, are today every more insistent and imperative. Andy Warhol already understood this tendency very well back in the seventies.

And New York restaurants now have a new thing — they don't sell their food, they sell their atmosphere. [...] They caught on that what people really care about is changing their atmosphere for a couple of hours. That's why they can get away with just selling their atmosphere with a minimum of actual food. Pretty soon when food prices go really up, they'll be selling only atmosphere. If people are really all that hungry, they can bring food with them when they go out to dinner, but otherwise, instead of "going out to dinner" they'll just be "going out to atmosphere." (Warhol 1975, 159)

The discipline that, better than any other, has intuited the potential of the atmospheric resource to condition the perception of places, and by extension people's attitudes — individual and collective — is marketing. Think, for example, of the activity of interior design in characterising a commercial space. As the philosopher Peter Sloterdijk notes, "air design aims at directly modifying the mood of airspace users — it serves the indirectly manifest purpose of [...] contributing to heightened product acceptance and willingness to buy." Atmosphere plays a crucial role: it "comes to have a central place as a 'discrete marketing instrument'" (2009, 94). In this perspective, the architectural setting of the point of sale becomes communication strategy and reinforcement of the link with the client, interfering with their capacity to evaluate the goods and their level of satisfaction (including the satisfaction of passing time inside the store). The atmospheric performance of commercial spaces, fruit of sensory and experiential marketing operations, fits perfectly in the "primary trend in consumer society towards a development of experience markets and 'scenes' in which atmospheres are made available as composite situations of stimuli, signs and chances for contact" (Sloterdijk 2016, 168).

The subject of atmosphere understood as constitutive character proves extremely valid and pertinent also if extended to urban landscapes (Hasse 2012). "The point is that cities have both things," clarifies the anthropologist Franco La Cecla. There are "an internal side, with the identity of belonging, and an external one, representing a wider scale, and the image imposed from outside" (2020, chapter III). The harmonized atmospheric effect of cities is unquestionable, regardless of whether it is perceived as positive or negative. Cities never have a neutral temperament: even in their anonymous way of being, vaunting a recognisable and describable identity. In some cases, atmosphere invokes remotely, for example through first-person accounts or commercial spots, it can be more exhaustive and fulfilling than direct experience *in situ*; this last is inevitably dirtied by distractions and limits exacted by reality, which dilute the general impression, weakening it with respect to how it has always been dreamed of. "Each city continues to express 'a special character, a slang or dialect, a form of humour, which sometimes has a special label,' in other words an atmosphere,"[30] confirms Tonino Griffero. "It is overall an image that works, no matter how impressionistic, prejudicial, metaphorical or even merely virtual it is, as in the case of city views only known through cinema" (2014a, 88). The skyline of Manhattan recapitulates all these observations in itself, becoming the most reproduced and imitated urban episode ever. In this continual reinterpretation, it inevitably undergoes simplifications that render its image stereotyped. The clichés, including from an atmospheric point of view, work in the following manner: they must be unambiguous and persuasive; they must offer desirable atmospheres in which to immerge and ideally project oneself. A synthesis of a few essential values is needed, which can even be intentionally designed.

On occasions, the atmosphere of an urban organism is so suggestive that one feels the need to repeat its overall configuration, with exaggerated accuracy. With the objective of relocating the much-loved French atmosphere in China, 2007 sees the completion of the building experiment of Tianducheng, a perfect Chinese replica of Parisian architecture, originally conceived as a deluxe area on the outskirts of Hangzhou, but long uninhabited. As seen in the provocative reportage *Paris Syndrome*[31] curated by the French photographer François Prost, in Tianducheng there are (extremely precise) copies of the Tour Eiffel, the *grands boulevards*, *hôtels particuliers* with typical mansard roofs, the old oil street lamps as well as fragments of the Château de Versailles. And yet, in this idealized Paris, apart from the architectural shapes, there is nothing of Paris: "it is completely lacking in atmosphere," explains the photographer, "because the Chinese of Tianducheng live as they do in any other place in China: they go to bed early, they get up early, they go for a walk at the weekend and immediately go back home, they practically only eat Chinese food."[32] Tianducheng is the

---

30 The internal quote refers to Rykwert 2000.
31 Prost, François. 2017. *Paris Syndrome*. The reportage is viewable online on the documentarist's site — www.francoisprost.com, last accessed 23 May 2021.
32 This is how François Prost describes the experience of the replica-city of Tianducheng in an interview for the magazine *Vanity Fair*. See Salsi, Fabiana. 2018. "Parigi: Sai riconoscere quella vera da quella falsa?" *Vanity Fair* (online), 21 February 2018, n.p. — www.vanityfair.it, last accessed 23 May 2021.

stereotype of atmospheric charisma par excellence, a vulgarization of its communicative function, a flattening of its potential. Personal representations, accredited by the daily experience of those who actually live in a particular urban space or constructed during spontaneous walks of situationist inspiration, such as the absent-minded *flâneur*, are quite another thing — another atmosphere.

Eighth node: atmosphere as aura

Atmosphere relates to the concept of aura, or rather the architectonic work's inherent character of oneness, which turns it into myth. This version of atmosphere introduces the interpretation of the notion of aura put forward by Walter Benjamin (1892–1940) in his critical essay *The Work of Art in the Age of Mechanical Reproduction*.[33]

> The uniqueness of a work of art is inseparable from its being imbedded in the fabric of tradition. This tradition itself is thoroughly alive and extremely changeable. An ancient statue of Venus, for example, stood in a different traditional context with the Greeks, who made it an object of veneration, than with the clerics of the Middle Ages, who viewed it as an ominous idol. Both of them, however, were equally confronted with its uniqueness, that is, its aura. (Benjamin 2007, 223)

The exclusive value accorded to the architectonic artefact, its aura, is tied to the cultural importance that it is given by the community (not only architectural): the edifice must be embraced in its quality of singular architecture, wrapped in a halo of originality and disciplinary authority. There are three requirements for us to be able to speak of an auratic prerogative. 1. — First requirement: *to be an architecture*, unequivocally accepted as such, and not an ordinary construction product. It is fundamental to distinguish between a (semantically autonomous) architectonic work and a building output (lacking artistic value, aimed at solving strictly structural aspects). The aesthetic experience transmitted by an architecture crosses the territory of technique and function, claiming its own specific semanticity, in other words its desire to communicate with people, to respond to their innate need for meanings, without limiting itself to finding

---

33 There are four versions of the essay: three in German (the first from 1935, which is entirely incorporated in the following two, the second entitled *Zweite Fassung* of 1936, and the third known as *Dritte Fassung* of 1939) and one in French (that came out in 1936, translated by Pierre Klossowski, with the final supervision of Benjamin himself); none of them can be considered the definitive or canonical version.

responses instrumental to their needs (Johnson 2002, 2015). As such, an architectonic opus "offers pleasurable shapes and surfaces moulded for the touch of the eye and other senses, but it also incorporates and integrates physical and mental structures, giving our existential experience a strengthened coherence and significance" (Pallasmaa 2012a, 13). 2. — Second requirement: the unrepeatable *character of singularity and originality*, or rather of uniqueness and authenticity, of the architectonic artefact; said character differentiates it from any copy, integral or partial, freed from the archetypical spatial-temporal location, in which the role of historical testimony of the primeval model resides. This issue takes us back to Walter Benjamin.

> Even the most perfect reproduction of a work of art is lacking in one element: its presence in time and space, its unique existence at the place where it happens to be. This unique existence of the work of art determined the history to which it was subject throughout the time of its existence. [...] The presence of the original is the prerequisite to the concept of authenticity. [...] [T]hat which withers in the age of mechanical reproduction is the aura of the work of art. (Benjamin 2007, 220–221)

Thus, every architectural composition must defend the objectual originality to which its historical root is anchored. 3. — Third (and last) requirement: the title of "unique and authentic architecture" must be *universally recognised*, validating the project as a certain and authoritative reference — most of all within its disciplinary field. Only in this way can its enchantment become a fully-fledged symbol that can be raised to myth.

The auratic halo of a given architectural work has often been identified in the particular atmosphere that the artefact is thought to be able to emanate — an atmosphere capable of evoking emotions, suggestions, and memories. Even at a semantic level, there is a consistent affinity between the words "aura" and "atmosphere," as demonstrated by the group of words "air/aura/atmosphere," widely used in the nineteenth century.[34] Steven Connor, professor of English language and literature at Cambridge University correlates the widespread and frequent use of the term "atmosphere" to its potential juxtaposition to the auratic essence: "the word 'atmosphere' came to be used more and more," indeed, "to express the qualities of specific

---

34   See "aria," in *Nuovo Dizionario dei Sinonimi della Lingua Italiana*. 1838. Ed. by N. Tommaseo, vol. I, item n. 236. Firenze: Gio Pietro Vieusseux. — "Aria/aura/aere/atmosfera" (50).

places or environments, according to the logic of the aura whereby a figure might be thought to exhale or extrude its own niche" (2010, 194). A link that the anthropologist Tim Ingold emphasizes: "there is a quite different sense in which the concept of atmosphere is commonly used [...]. It has to do with the evocation of feeling, and is roughly equivalent to what Walter Benjamin called 'aura'" (2012, 79). Gernot Böhme puts forward a perceptual take on aura in the space-time interplay, reaffirming that the aura, understood in the Benjamin's meaning of the word, "is clearly something which flows forth spatially, almost something like a breath or a haze — precisely an atmosphere" (1993, 117). He goes on to comment that "to perceive aura is to absorb it into one's own bodily state of being" and that "what is perceived is an indeterminate spatially extended quality of feeling" (Böhme, 117–118).

Furthermore, it is important to make clear that the auratic condition of atmosphere presupposes immediate recognition, all the more automatic the more relevant the value of the architectonic work or the more famous the name of the architect. This last observation is shown to be true above all in contemporary times, when an unprecedented politico-mediatic cult of authorship has transformed internationally famed architects into veritable icons for society. The family of modern starchitects produces gurus that dictate modes and tendencies, colonizing magazine covers, television programmes, social media, and advertising campaigns (Lo Ricco and Micheli, 2003). A large number of designers has turned into lucrative Warholian machines of atmosphere, featuring aura. Atmosphere is sold, aura is bought.

> Some company recently was interested in buying my "aura." They didn't want my product. They kept saying, "We want your aura." I never figured out what they wanted. But they were willing to pay a lot for it. So then I thought that if somebody was willing to pay that much for my it, I should try to figure out what it is. I think "aura" is something that only somebody else can see, and they only see as much of it as they want to. It's all in the other person's eyes.
> (Warhol 1975, 77)

Ninth node: atmosphere as collector of memories

Atmosphere is intrinsically tied to the personal experience of the individual, of whom it condenses the intimate experiences and mental free associations. The relationship between the atmospheric dynamics and the temporal dimension is extremely intense, particularly on a level of subjective sensitivity. Human beings live "in mental worlds, in which the material, the experienced, the remembered and the imagined completely fuse into each other" (Pallasmaa 2002, 18). The exchanges with memory, sudden and for the most part nonconscious, provoke temporal swings of cognition, both backwards and forwards with respect to the instant present in which the emotional stimulus is activated. Tonino Griffero clarifies this when he affirms that atmospheres "undoubtedly depend also on the co-perception of past and expected atmospheres that are not in act." An example makes it clearer: "the atmosphere of a hospital is tense precisely because we anticipate the situation to follow (the visit, the diagnosis, etc.) and we remember earlier ones (further waits, etc.)" (2014c, 37).

The action of memory can derive from an act of will that is aware and deliberate, or — as more often occurs in atmospheric contagion — it can be an instinctive reflex that is beyond the subject's control. In the first case, by means of a series of fragmentary images, suggested by memory, atmosphere constructs a scenario parallel to physical reality, a poetic transposition of the permanent memory, which replicates excerpts taken from the personal repertory of knowledge of the world. Examples are all those settings that, from the initial design step, are meant to evoke familiar atmospheres, such as our own home, childhood retreats, and special places. Here, the atmospheric swarm is primed by the sense of belonging, safety, and confidence, whispered by our past. Consider the private universe of the bedroom: "the bedroom is a box that is both real and imaginary," writes Michelle Perrot. "Like a sacrament, closing the door protects the privacy of the group, the couple, or the person" (2018, 2–3). Each detail contributes to the building of a condensed world, where the atmosphere is the representation of the personal microcosm. "Every bedroom is more or less a 'cabinet of curiosities' [...]: albums, photographs, posters, souvenirs brought back from travels [...]. Anything can be included in these miniature models of the world" (Perrot, 3).

Whereas, in the second case the transition to long-term memory occurs in an accidental and totally involuntary way. This happens, as per psychology textbooks,[35] when the stimulus is high intensity or is characterised by a large discrepancy with respect to the person's usual experiences. Without warning or intent, the emotional impulse is triggered that radiates an atmospheric tension, capable of bringing together the individual with their architectonic surroundings. Memory reinterprets the

---

35 See § "long-term memory" (chapter IV), in Canestrari, Renzo, and Godino, Antonio. 2002. *Introduzione alla Psicologia Generale*. Milano: Bruno Mondadori.

space, assigning new meanings. Memory is never the exact copy of the lived experience, but is effectively an affective portrayal of it. Namely, spatial experience is revisited and rebuilt on the basis of the emotions that we felt and still feel.

The design psychologist Sally Augustin (Augustin 2009; Augustin and Coleman 2012) points out how in establishing an emotional tie with the spaces they use, human beings are more likely to form attachments with places that reflect something of their individual story and to which, therefore, they confer greater value — such as the area where they grew up or the field on which they regularly played sport. People can also feel emotional attachment to places where they have never been before but that hold a certain importance for their social extraction or cultural background. A stubborn sense of disorientation and displeasure accompanies every hypothesis or resolution to alter those places, as though a part of the person were damaged or even erased. "While we prefer to be in familiar-type spaces," observes Augustin, "we don't want environments to be completely static; our moods, for example, are best when spaces slowly and gradually evolve from one form to another" (2017, 62).

The atmospheric potential of memory, an agent as much for "habituation extended in time" as for "shock" (Neutra 1954, 229), induces an emotional-affective involvement, which is directly proportional to the level of acuteness and vividness of the inveterate memory. For Juhani Pallasmaa, between novelty and echoes of the past, it is the latter that wins, all the more when they allude to intimate questions of the subject.

> There are fabricated images in today's architecture and art that are flat and without an emotional echo, but there are also novel images that resonate with remembrance. The latter are at the same time mysterious and familiar, obscure and clear. They move us through the remembrances and associations, emotions and empathy that they awaken in us. Artistic novelty can move us only provided it touches something that we already possess in our very being. Every profound artistic work surely grows from memory, not from rootless intellectual invention. (Pallasmaa 2009b, 38)

The emotional tone of the atmospheric reaction depends on that of the situation brought to light by the memory. Sensory stimuli play a decisive role in the triggering of memory. "Every architectural setting," it is useful to remember, "has its auditive, haptic, olfactory, and even hidden gustatory qualities, and those properties give the visual percept its sense of fullness and life" (Pallasmaa 2011b, 52). The mnesic strength of an atmospheric connection is the result of a sensory dialogue, in which the voice of the olfactory sense stands out significantly. "Another way to take up more space is with perfume," states Andy Warhol (1975, 150). "Of the five senses, smell has the closest thing to the full power of the past. [...] Seeing, hearing, touching, tasting are just not as powerful as smelling if you want your whole being to go back for a second to something" (Warhol, 151). It is enough to fleetingly sniff an aroma to be projected to the exact moment in which that olfactory accent was created, to be taken back to its place of origin. Likewise, one can simply divert their attention for the rapture of the memory to cease. "The good thing about a smell-memory is that the feeling of being transported stops the instant you stop smelling, so there are no after effects." As Andy Warhol confides, "it's a neat way to reminisce" (1975, 151).

The spatial experience is, often, mainly played out on a visual exploration of its components:[36] and yet, however many — innumerable — times one might have observed a place, in real life or portrayed in images, however familiar or conventional that place may be, the fulfilment of the glance, whether wandering and poetic or vigilant and rational, can never produce the same emotional tremor that perfume or a bad smell can impart. Tonino Griffero, who emphasizes the primacy of *orosensory atmospheres* (that is, based on the oral sensory unity given by smell and taste), illustrates the distinctive mechanisms involved. "Unlike other sensibles, taste and smell are not easily communicable, they cannot be willingly recalled nor can they be suppressed for long and intentionally through their organs (nose and mouth), because survival itself is at stake" (2014a, 68 n. 41). Although hard to express, since they are extremely personal and tenaciously uncontrollable, olfactory suggestions allow us to elaborate descriptions of sincere and detailed experienced places. In the words of Andy Warhol (for whose dialectic I now feel a certain affection, as the many quotes suggest) the fresh and excited atmosphere of his city of adoption, New York, is evoked through its smells and memories, or better still, memories of its

---

[36] "We are visually dominant creatures. That is, we all mostly tend to think, reason, and imagine visually" (Spence 2020, 2). Although we have to learn from the growing critique of the ocularcentric obsession of contemporary architecture and affirm the crucial relevance of a multisensory approach, we recognize that "there is also a need to understand vision more profoundly and through multiple lenses" (Pérez Liebergesell, Vermeersch, and Heylighen 2019, 47).

smells. One can quite clearly make Manhattan out in its numerous aspects, even with one's eyes closed.

When I'm walking around New York I'm always aware of the smells around me: the rubber mats in office buildings; upholstered seats in movie theaters; pizza; Orange Julius; espresso-garlic-oregano; burgers; dry cotton tee-shirts; neighborhood grocery stores; chic grocery stores; the hot dogs and sauerkraut carts; hardware store smell; stationery store smell; souvlaki; the leather and rugs at Dunhill, Mark Cross, Gucci; the Moroccan-tanned leather on the street-racks; new magazines, back-issue magazines; typewriter stores; Chinese import stores (the mildew from the freighter); India import stores; Japanese import stores; record stores; health food stores; soda-fountain drugstores; cut-rate drugstores; barber shops; beauty parlors; delicatessens; lumber yards; the wood chairs and tables in the N.Y. Public Library; the donuts, pretzels, gum, and grape soda in the subways; kitchen appliance departments; photo labs; shoe stores; bicycle stores; the paper and printing inks in Scribner's, Brentano's, Doubleday's, Rizzoli, Marboro, Bookmasters, Barnes & Noble; shoe-shine stands; grease-batter; hair pomade; the good cheap candy smell in the front of Woolworth's and the dry-goods smell in the back; the horses by the Plaza Hotel; bus and truck exhaust; architects' blueprints; cumin, fenugreek, soy sauce, cinnamon; fried platanos; the train tracks in Grand Central Station; the banana smell of dry cleaners; exhausts from apartment house laundry rooms; East Side bars (creams); West Side bars (sweat); newspaper stands; record stores; fruit stands in all the different seasons — strawberry, watermelon, plum, peach, kiwi, cherry, Concord grape, tangerine, murcot, pineapple, apple — and I love the way the smell of each fruit gets into the rough wood of the crates and into the tissue-paper wrappings. (Warhol 1975, 152–153)

Anyone could compile a list like this one — a list that turns into the emotional seismograph of a hermetically intimate atmosphere, ignited by memories that are concatenated at the level of sensory sensations.

Tenth node: atmosphere as perceptive experience

Atmosphere is the emotional-perceptive tension between the architectural qualities of a space and the subjective sensitivity of the spatially immersed individual. It is a condition that is all but metaphorical or spiritual. Rather, it is a physical phenomenon that emerges from the physicality of the architectonic elements that make up the context and the physicality of the bodies that dynamically interact with it. Two poles are essential: perceiving subject and architectonically organized, and as a consequence characterised, space. "Taking possession of space is the first gesture of living things, of men and of animals, of plants and of clouds, a fundamental manifestation of equilibrium and of duration," teaches Le Corbusier; it follows that "the release of esthetic emotion is a special function of space" (1948, 7). Human beings take possession of the space, occupying it through their own body; and, through their own body, they know and interpret that space. "The bodily emotions we experience in considering an architectural work," as the art historian Heinrich Wölfflin theorized at the end of the nineteenth century, "cannot be denied" ([1886] 1994, 154). They are the product of a complex process of assimilation and metabolisation of received stimuli, which involves several of the body's senses simultaneously.[37] Atmospheric contact is established at the moment in which a *sensory imbalance* arises, when on the emotional level there takes place "a certain, variously qualified, modification of the corporeal space, of the sensed space" (Griffero 2005a, 293).

Or, in other words, faced with an environment that changes, it transpires that it is the emotions allowing us to modify our intentions and our behaviour; it is the emotions that fashion the general atmosphere of the context and discipline its impact on our perception; it is the emotions that institute a psychophysiological relationship between the subject and their architectonic surroundings. In this particular understanding of the concept of atmosphere, certainly the least figurative expression of all,[38] it is implicit that the emotions should be understood in their pre-eminently biological sense: they are, namely, somatic events, electrochemical trails, which regulate the reaction of the organism confronted with external input by means of automatic acts of evaluation. They are biophysical responses. In this context, there are those who — like Juhani Pallasmaa (2016b) — even promote a definition of atmosphere as "sixth human sense" (2013, 55). Furthermore, he puts forward an update of the list of *multiple intelligences*, styled by the American psychologist Howard Gardner (1999), who rejects single decoding of intelligence as a cerebral category. Alongside

---

37 "Human multisensory perception is the result of synthesis and successive abstractions, which integrate the information deriving from single senses in a space-time continuum" (Buiatti 2014, 19).
38 Equally, although from another point of view, to that of atmo-technologies for the optimization of air quality: cf. the section "atmosphere as microclimate" (first node). The term "atmo-technologies" is used by the philosopher Peter Sloterdijk. It indicates the experimental techniques used for microclimatic control of the air, without which "modern forms of existence in urban or rural contexts would be unimaginable" (2009, 92).

the previously accredited types,[39] Pallasmaa flanks four further varieties (2015, 61–62), among which are *emotional intelligence* and *atmospheric intelligence*.

The role that architectural design plays with regard to the modulation of atmospheric potential is considerable and — above all — inevitable. Atmosphere that determines the experience of space "constitutes other surfaces, other grounds, other ceilings," points out Le Corbusier ([1930] 2015, 77). Physical bodies afford incessant emotional invitations. Such impulses are, however, so closely interconnected to each other that they cannot always be traced back to a specific material source. To influence the emotivity of someone occupying a space, we need an all-inclusive atmosphere, capable of rendering a space atmospherically perceptible in its indissoluble complexity. "The visitor and user, the customer and the patient are all touched or moved by these atmospheres. The architect, however, creates them, more or less consciously," states Gernot Böhme. "The sensual items which he posits: the colours, the design of surfaces, the lines, the arrangements and the constellations are, at the same time a physiognomy from which the atmosphere emanates" (1991, 36). Analysis of the so-called "generators of atmosphere" (Böhme 2013b, 27), or rather of those factors that more than others contribute to composing the atmospheric sense and conditioning the spatial perception of the agents, is today the object of numerous interdisciplinary studies.[40] By coordinating the specialist knowledge of different scientific sectors (for example psychology, psychiatry, and neuroscience), they lay the foundations for drawing up design guidelines, directed at intervening in specific areas, such as those dedicated to the medical treatment of particular clinical populations or social-healthcare for old people. One thinks of *milieu therapy*, the aim of which is to enhance the therapeutic power that the health facility acquires as part of the cure itself (Martin, Nettleton, and Buse 2019): in such a context, we investigate the development of the atmosphere of an environment to improve the mental and physical conditions of the user/patient. In this case, atmosphere assumes the features of catalyst of *psychophysical well-being*.

It is interesting to observe how artistic research has for a long time been exploring the atmospheric dimension, mainly attracted by the nature

---

39 Logical-mathematical, verbal-linguistic, visual-spatial, bodily-kinaesthetic, musical, interpersonal, intrapersonal, naturalistic, ethical, and existential intelligences.
40 This topic is discussed in more detail in the fifth chapter. See the fourth subchapter "The Polyphony of the Senses," section "first property: atmosphere is composite."

of being "'in-between' of a reality so often presupposed as dualistic (subject/object)" (Pérez-Gómez 2016, 32). In promoting the proliferation and circulation of aesthetic emotions, atmospheres become the *tool of interaction*: interaction between the visitor and the staged set, between visitor and artist, between visitor and other visitors. In short: between bodies and spatial qualities. I find it is helpful to consider some episodes taken from the world of contemporary art, given that — by exaggerating experimentation on perceptual mechanisms — it renders them clearer and so more comprehensible. In the encounter of art and atmosphere, one of the most illustrious precursors is the master of light James Turrell, born in Los Angeles in 1943. From the late sixties, Turrell created a vast universe of works, which offer intense revelations on the perception of the luminous phenomenon and its capacities to become solid matter. He was joined on this research itinerary by colleague Robert Irwin and by the perception psychologist Edward Wortz, both members of the American movement Light and Space. James Turrell's installations, celebrating the visual and emotional effects of light, shape sophisticated atmospheric spaces that are anything but static and inscrutable.

To explore the emotional-perceptive essence of atmospheric bliss, the artist has perfected a wide range of design models.[41] There are the *Ganzfeld* (a German term translatable as "complete field"), in which Turrell tests a surreal technique of sensory deprivation, based on the total loss of perception of depth: such a result is obtained through the controlled use of light and the shaping of the space by means of rounded corners and sloping surfaces. "The effect of a Ganzfeld can be compared to that of a snow storm, when it becomes impossible to distinguish clearly what you are seeing before you."[42] There are the *Shallow Spaces*, a linear or angular development, in which — with mirror effects that flatten the space while three-dimensional rendering deconstructs and dilates it — Turrell crowns light as an unrestrained substance generating spatiality. Light effects trace elementary geometric shapes, with clear cuts and in primary colours, but the game of optical illusions realized reflects contradictory perceptions: light, by altering and manipulating space, distorts it. And the spectator, fully immersed in its intangible presence, is hypnotized and disoriented — warmed or cooled by the sensations aroused in them. Then there are the

---

41   See Adcock 1990; Sambonet 1998; Noever 2001; Govan and Kim 2013.
42   James Turrell's description of the Ganzfeld set up in the Scuderia Grande at Villa Panza, Varese (2013–2019) — www.aisthesis-fai.it, last accessed 25 May 2021.

Tunnel Pieces, corridors of light and colour, that can be explored freely. Movement mixes with visual dizziness and produces a pure, alienating perceptual experience.

There are many more examples worth citing. I shall conclude with the most ambitious project of all, launched over forty years ago. Back in 1977, James Turrell bought an extinct volcano in northern Arizona: the *Roden Crater*.[43] Nestled in the arid region of the Painted Desert, the site — apparently uncontaminated — shows no sign of its sophisticated internal modelling, an intarsia of underground rooms, purposely designed to capture natural light, which only enters at certain hours of the day and specific seasons of the year. The structure is an observatory designed for the contemplation of celestial phenomena, in which to combine scientific experiments and artistic projects based on light, mixing the two. Harry Francis Mallgrave describes it thus:

> Turrell's chthonic project [...] promises to be one of the more elaborate and primal investigations of atmospheric perception or "wordless thought" ever undertaken, one in which the artist, in his long-standing quest to reduce light to tactile values, seeks "to play a music of the spheres in light." Architects are generally not trained to approach the issue of light or atmosphere with such epiphanic intensity, but they can certainly appreciate the notion of light having both tactile and material values. (Mallgrave 2013, 158)

Eleventh node: atmosphere as mood

Atmosphere is identified in the pervasive emotional charge that is radiated by a space and can influence the mood of anyone relating with that spatiality. "Every space, place and situation is tuned in a specific way, and it projects an atmosphere promoting distinct moods and feelings," explains Juhani Pallasmaa. "We live in resonance with our world, and architecture mediates this very resonance" (2014b, 76). A word that sums up the entire process is *Stimmung*. The German word is so complex that it is very hard to define or translate. The concept "covers three phenomena," which are "harmony, mood, and atmosphere" (Krebs 2014, 1257), and is interpretable as subjective state of mind "infused" in the body of architecture and the landscape (Krebs, 1258) — or rather: a diffuse atmosphere, an aesthetic experience, of which we resound and appropriate its transmitted sensations. In philosophical literature the notion of atmosphere was frequently

---

43 See De Rosa 2007.

associated with that of *Stimmung* (Bille, Bjerregaard, and Sørensen 2015): Martin Heidegger ([1927] 1962), Otto Friedrich Bollnow (1941), Leo Spitzer (1942a, 1942b), Hubertus Tellenbach (1968, 1981), and Gernot Böhme (1993, 1995a) are some of the authors who have looked into the nature of atmosphere as a link between perceiving subject and architectonic context, recognizing in sensory and emotional experience a role of crucial importance.

When we explore the atmospheric dynamic in its meaning of "mood," accepting it both as a combination of constant qualities of temperament and, more often, as a transitory attitude, the fulcrum of the question is moved mainly to the subject; which is to say: to their point of view, to their affective sensitivity, and to their tendency to interact with the instinctive and involuntary emotions provoked by the surrounding environment. Obviously, the influence of this last does not disappear, but the perspective from which the attuning mechanisms are observed is decentralized. The universe of *Stimmung* does, indeed, inspire "the world of 'natural' harmony between movements of the emotions and the presence of things" (Baudrillard 1996, 24). In other words, it implies bilateral perception. "We may touch objects, or not. They, in turn, may touch us (or not), and they may be experienced either as imposing or inconsequential," specifies Hans Ulrich Gumbrecht. "Atmospheres and moods include the physical dimension of phenomena" (2012, 6). The emotional tones imbuing objects and spaces populated by them produce atmospheres, in which anyone occupying those spaces remains immersed and permeated. Sustained by the vague (but penetrating) sense of a perception, atmospheric *Stimmungen* turn out to be extremely hazy and labyrinthine personal experiences. They mark out psychological territories, dug and shaped by inner forces, which sometimes coincide with physical spaces reserved for one's intimacy, in which to isolate oneself to listen and tune to own existential emotions.

> The desire for personal space is relatively universal; it is found across civilizations and historical eras. Sleep, sex, love, sickness, prayer, meditation, reading, writing — the needs of the body but also of the soul compel us to retreat to our own rooms, which may take many forms. Caves and huts, cells and corners, the boat cabin, the train compartment, the enclosed horse-drawn carriage — we have been unimaginably ingenious in devising ways to hide ourselves away. (Perrot 2018, 57)

Frank Lloyd Wright, who liked to be known as an "architect of atmosphere" (Wigley 1998a, 18), was firmly convinced that a person's individual nature was influenced by the atmospheric temperament of the space they lived in: "whether people are conscious of this or not," annotates Wright, "they actually derive countenance and sustenance from the 'atmosphere' of the things they live in or with" (1954, 135). Thus defined, atmospheric impact leads to an extremely *introvert subjectivity*, an intimate way of feeling, impossible to analyse rationally or to measure: only the perceiving agent can (try to) describe the felt experience, out of a thousand uncertainties and imprecisions. Peter Zumthor, for example, is ambiguous when he explains the affective importance of architectural atmospheres, speaking about "this singular density and mood, this feeling of presence, well-being, harmony, beauty… under whose spell I experience what I otherwise would not experience in precisely this way" (as cited in Anderson 2014, 154).

Deconstructing and recomposing these inner landscapes, built on personal sensations, emotional states, and mood tones, we can sketch changing geographies, or better, one might say *psychogeographical narrations,* if we take up the theories of psychoaffective transport put forward by the Situationists. In the first issue of the *Internationale Situationniste*, published in June 1958, psychogeographical practice was introduced as the "study of the specific effects of the geographical environment (whether consciously organized or not) on the emotions and behavior of individuals" (Knabb 2006, 52). Dismantling the consolidated topographical schemes of urban planning and rejecting the conventions imposed by society, which dictate rules on how to live the city, both for entertainment and necessity, a psychogeographical approach affirms itself through the exercise of *spatial dérive* ("drifting").[44] It encourages one to get lost in contexts, familiar or not, letting oneself be pulled along by the current of one's own perceptions, which follow spontaneously on each other. The experience of drifting requires an ability to wander aimlessly and without restrictions of time.

> In a *dérive* one or more persons during a certain period drop their relations, their work and leisure activities, and all their other usual motives for movement and action, and let themselves be drawn by the attractions of the terrain and the encounters they find there. Chance is a less important factor in this activity than one might think: from a *dérive* point of view cities have psychogeographical contours, with constant currents, fixed

---

44 "One of the basic Situationist practices is the *dérive*, a technique of rapid passage through varied ambiences" — excerpt from *Internationale Situationniste* 2 (1958), as translated in Knabb 2006, 62.

points and vortexes that strongly discourage entry into or exit from certain zones. (Knabb 2006, 62)

The aim of the psychogeographical dynamics is clear: "spatial development must take the affective realities [...] into account" (Debord [1957] 2002, 44). There follows the possibility of a new manner of understanding and living the urban ecosystem: "a new architecture, a free architecture [...] will not play at first on free, poetic lines and forms [...] but rather on the atmospheric effects of rooms, corridors, streets, atmospheres linked to the behaviors they contain" (Debord, 45). In this way, urban organisms are subverted, thrown into disarray, and sorted into archipelagos of emotional clots: so-called *unities of atmosphere* and *dwellings*[45] emerge, presented in the second issue of the journal *Internationale Situationniste* (1958). An operation of affective resignification is carried out, in which the emotions arbitrarily rescript zones of attraction or repulsion. The enormous potential offered by atmospheric sensitivity becomes for the Situationists not only an opportunity for urban transformation, but also the innovative motor for social discussion. Atmosphere evolves into the stimulator of awareness. "Atmosphere becomes the basis of political action," sustains Mark Wigley, describing New Babylon[46] — the Situationist nomad utopia — as a "huge atmosphere jukebox." "The seemingly ephemeral is mobilized as the agent of concrete struggle," he explains (1998b, 13).

3. *Interweaving*

In the absence of an exact and unambiguous definition, I have tried to clarify an imprecise term through an overview of equally imprecise terms such as *identity, imagination, character, aura*, and *Stimmung*. One might object that it is not necessary to develop lists such as this one, getting caught — as often happens — "in the illusion that semantic clarification passes through the proliferation of (physical and spiritual) meanings of [a] term" (Griffero 2020a, 141). In truth, aware of the instability of the atmospheric subject and its slippery multiformity, I wanted to establish a form of organisation for the inquiry that would help me to find my way through

---

45 "Today the different unities of atmosphere and of dwellings are not precisely marked off, but are surrounded by more or less extended bordering regions" (Knabb 2006, 66).
46 The project of a nomadic camp, on a planetary scale, ideated by the Situationist artist Constant Nieuwenhuys (1920–2005).

the nebulous domain of atmospheric existence. I compiled a pilot book that, however fragmentary, was scrupulously studied for the architectural discipline: it outlines the prevalent flows that innervate the atmospheric dynamics, indicating the possible routes to travel — an operation that is almost indispensable to begin navigation. Often one has the impression that a selected meaning might be assigned to another category too, undergoing an alternative and complementary interpretative recall. In other words: if an atmospheric impulse reveals itself above all as feeling effused in a space, it does not imply the exclusion, for example, of mnemonic trails or metaphorical associations, rather it suggests the opposite.

It is in the penultimate meaning (*atmosphere as perceptive experience*, as a condition for emotional resonance) that this research work plants the seed for its personal interpretation of atmosphere.

IV
ATMOSPHERIC REVIVAL

1. *Evolutionary Background*

In the beginning was Heidegger. Martin Heidegger is reputedly "the discoverer of world-disclosing moods in the philosophical context": an attribution given him by the German philosopher Peter Sloterdijk (2016, 674). Through the audacious trilogy, *Sphären* (literally "Spheres"),[1] published between 1998 and 2004, Sloterdijk builds an original theory of space, based on the centrality of the atmospheric condition. By means of the atmospheric filter he experiments with a philosophical-cultural redefinition of the contemporary era and its multifocal relationship with the real, as we see above all in the third volume, *Schäume* ("Foams"). "We begin to understand that man is not only what he eats, but what he breathes and that in which he is immersed" (Sloterdijk 2009, 84).[2] In the following extract, Professor Sloterdijk sums up the evolutionary trajectory that the atmospheric phenomenon has gone through in the modern era.

> Because atmospheres are non-concrete and non-informative by nature (and did not seem controllable), they were passed over by the ancient and modern European culture of reason on its long road to the objectification and informatization of all things and facts. [...] Factual sciences and discourse theories alike refused to admit that something could exist apart from the *words* and the *things*, something that was neither of these yet more expansive, earlier and more pervasive than both. The nineteenth century did attempt to grasp this subtle third element when it spoke of *milieu* or *ambiente*, while the twentieth provided its own version by translating it into *Umwelt* and *environment*; none of these concepts succeeded in capturing the atmospheric component, however,

---

1   The three volumes are respectively entitled *Blasen* ("Bubbles" — Microspherology), *Globen* ("Globes" — Macrospherology), and *Schäume* ("Foams" — Plural Spherology).
2   The book *Terror from the Air* (2009) constitutes a sort of introductory appendix to the third volume of the collection, *Foams* (2016).

and the sole progress was from dull to duller. [...] When modern philosophy — fundamental ontology in particular — returned from its two-thousand-year exile in the supersensible and began to re-establish its rooting in being-in-the-world, it rightly described *mood* as the first opening up of existence to the why and wherefore of the world. One could view Heidegger's early work as the Magna Carta of a previously unattempted onto-climatology. (Sloterdijk 2014, 137–138: original italics)

"It could be that we now devote more attention to atmospheres," notes Hans Ulrich Gumbrecht, "than fifty, two hundred, or five hundred years ago" (2012, 7). In fact, "atmosphere," "a word that sounded pompous in the 1930s," remarks Bruno Latour, "has now become commonplace, perhaps reflecting a universal condition" (2003, 29). In any case, it is in the first half of the twentieth century that the atmospheric ferment starts to slowly, hazily simmer. "In the period between the two wars, European culture begins to feel the growing need for atmospheric concepts, which can express the epochal changes in perception of communal space and ambience" (Carnevali 2006, 121). The philosophical machine is the first to get underway in search of answers. "The concept of 'atmosphere' is at the basis of a new philosophical orientation, which has its roots in the traditions of twentieth century phenomenology," explains Elisabetta Di Stefano, "and draws on both the line leading from Husserl to Merleau-Ponty and the phenomenological anthropology of Rothacker, Klages, and Hermann Schmitz" (2012, 14 n. 31). The explorative impetus is triggered with the greatest dynamism in Germany. In particular, one of the most important contributions (and, above all, more functional to this course of analysis) is consolidated in Neue Phänomenologie (New Phenomenology, in English), the philosophical current framed in the sixties by Hermann Schmitz (2019). It concerns, comments Tonino Griffero, "a theoretical project that, fully congruent with the actual rebirth of global scientific interest in the emotional, thinks of philosophy as a reflection of how 'one feels' in a certain space" (2014d, 162–163).

The atmospheric thought, incubated in the theoretical premises of Hermann Schmitz's New Phenomenology, and increasingly anchored to the theory of perception,[3] matures in the aesthetics research of Gernot Böhme, which contributes to promoting a New Aesthetics (1993). From a methodological point of view, therefore, the study of atmospheres has been

---

3 Picking up the aesthetics work of Alexander Gottlieb Baumgarten (Di Stefano 2012, 14 n. 31).

dominated — and is largely still dominated — by a phenomenological approach (or, to be more precise, neo-phenomenological), which from its German origin knew a vigorous resonance on an international level.[4] In parallel, the first disciplinarily autonomous steps were taken in the architectural field too. It was inevitable that from the start there would be involvement of the architectural bailiwick, insofar as it is the art and science of manipulating space, from the moment that "the notion of atmosphere always concerns a spatial sense of ambiance" (Böhme 1998, 112). Peter Sloterdijk registers the developments that, in the modern era, have fed the attraction between architectural production and atmospheric sensitivity.

As far as the architects of modernity are concerned, they not only became aware of their responsibility for the psychological comfort of a housing unit — one recalls Le Corbusier's concept of "psychic ventilation" — but also increasingly understood that in addition to the visible architectural structure, their product also had an atmospheric reality with an intrinsic value. The true dwelling space is an air sculpture traversed by its inhabitants like a breathable installation. [...] To the extent that buildings are thought of as spatial-plastic entities once more, there is a keener sense of the cavities (*les creux*) as autonomous realities demanding to be shaped. And just as the hothouses since the nineteenth century have been built purely for the sake of the climate that is meant to exist inside them, a number of the most important masters of spatial production in the twentieth converted to an explicit air and climate art. (Sloterdijk 2016, 526)

2. *Atmospheric Turn*

The present, that by convention can be approximated to the start of the third millennium, is seeing an agitated *spatial turn*, a shift in paradigm that seems "to have struck all the human sciences, suddenly once more interested in valorising a concrete and qualitatively articulated space rather than the natural science's abstract and isotropic space" (Griffero 2015, 156–157). And, more specifically, we can advance the hypothesis that there is an *atmospheric turn* in play: the first to speak of this was the German philosopher and chemist Jens Soentgen (Griffero 2014a; Gandy 2017) in 1998. Soentgen found the emergence in Europe of a new aesthetic-experiential fervour, germinated around the key notion of atmosphere, which at the close of the twentieth century provoked the phenomenological training ground, to then animate other areas of research such as cultural

---

4 In Italy, Tonino Griffero is the precursor and reference for the atmospheric frontier.

geography, anthropology, psychology, literature, and architecture. Tonino Griffero interprets this atmospheric turn as part of a more general *affective turn*,[5] developed in the humanities from the nineties, in favour of an emotional reading of reality: progressively the interest began to coagulate around the understanding of "the vague but expressive qualia of reality (its pathic 'how')" rather than "its quantified materiality or defined semantic value (its gnostic 'what')" (Griffero 2020c, 12). The affective turn "was born from the ashes of the linguistic one (and its hermeneutic and semiotic ramifications)," explains Griffero, "also resulting from the failure of both the deceptive cognitivist primacy and the omni-explicative model of data processing" (2020c, 16). One might ask if this "fast-career concept" of atmosphere (Griffero and Moretti 2018, 11) is only a short-term cultural tendency or if it is fuelled by deeper instances (Griffero 2019). What is certain is that today it "may even appear somewhat inflated" (Griffero 2020c, 16).

An immediate and notable inclination for interdisciplinary discussion stands out (De Matteis et al. 2019; Osler and Szanto 2021) — a predisposition for contaminations and synergies between profiles of different fields. One of the first encounters that formalized research on the atmospheric phenomenon under a design perspective in an academic setting is emblematic in this sense: the conference *Atmospheres, Architecture and Urban Space: New Conceptions of Management and the Social*,[6] held on 17 May 2011, and organised by the Copenhagen Business School (CBS), involved a philosopher (Gernot Böhme), a professor of political sociology (Christian Borch, who was the scientific coordinator), an artist (Olafur Eliasson), and an architect (Juhani Pallasmaa); four highly active exponents in today's panorama of study on the atmospheric dynamics, each from a different disciplinary sector and whose connection was not initially certain. The architecture debate convincingly supports this "turn towards (or perhaps a return to) atmospheric qualities" (Borch 2014, 7), both on a theoretical level and that of practical implementation. Obviously, "this is not to suggest that all architecture today revolves around atmospheric

---

5   "The urgency of today's new theories of resonance [...] is certainly not due to some mystical backlash but to a basic intellectual 'atmosphere' closely linked to the so-called 'affective turn' in the humanities" (Griffero 2020b, 95).

6   The experience fostered by the conference constitutes the programmatic premise of the volume *Architectural Atmospheres: On the Experience and Politics of Architecture* (Borch 2014), with which it shares the aim of encouraging investigation into atmospheres as much on an architectural as on a social theory level.

dimensions" (Borch, 7), but there is, without doubt, a tendency — constantly on the increase, albeit in different forms and with varied aims and results — to probe the atmospheric dimension.

In wanting (and needing) to find a shared significant debut for the renewed atmospheric aesthetics in the architectural field, I have established as *year zero* that of the launch of the book-manifesto *Atmospheres* by the Swiss architect Peter Zumthor, published for the first time in 2006.[7] Although it is a modest volume, of less than eighty pages, half of which are reserved for (decidedly poetic and powerful) images, and lacking explicit doctrinal claims, the text won over the architectural community, probably thanks in part to its delicate accessibility and expressive openness.[8] The main merit of this volume is that it stresses, for the first time and from the very title itself, the autonomy of the concept of atmosphere, without periphrasis or metaphor. Confirming its full dignity and integrity. "The title *Atmospheres* is generated by a question that has interested me for quite some time," begins Zumthor. "This is something we all know about," he emphasises (2006, 11).

Listening to Peter Zumthor, we are focusing on an apparently clear, intelligible, almost obvious question; in reality, this question is intrinsically complex, as we've tried to show in the previous chapters of this journey. It is important to note that the question has been raised by one of the most renowned architects on the international scene, in the very years in which his media exposure grows due to his winning the Pritzker Architecture Prize. It is 2009 — the year of the inversion, the reversal of direction: from that moment the tendency is to prefer for the assignment of this meaningful

---

7   The volume originated from a lecture held by Peter Zumthor on 1 June 2003, at the music and literature festival *Wege durch das Land* organised at the castle of Wendlinghausen in Germany.

8   It is interesting to note the results extrapolated from a survey launched in November 2017 by Davide Tommaso Ferrando and Sara Favargiotti, as part of the research project *Little Italy*, dedicated to the analysis of the new cultural and professional trends that distinguish the generation of Italian architects born in the eighties. A hundred and twenty candidates took part in the study, singly and collectively. It emerged that, with regard to fundamental reference texts for the construction of their own critical-design imaginary, the book *Atmospheres* by Peter Zumthor — not exactly a theoretical paper — was the fourth most cited contribution (preceded by *Delirious New York* and *S,M,L,XL* by Rem Koolhaas and *Weak and Diffuse Modernity* by Andrea Branzi). All the findings collected can be consulted on the online platform Are.na (www.are.na/little-italy/the-survey).

prize figures who, programmatically, reject the status of starchitect, supporters of a newfound aesthetics, that prevails as an antidote to that of the high-flown performance architecture, intensely commercialised during the first decade of the third millennium (Canepa 2018). There is a frenzied rediscovery of a sensibility tied to atmospheric transport, ignored for a long time, diminished in the role of perception phenomenon. Today, just to think about overlooking the effects of the involvement exercised by architectural atmospheres might seem far-fetched. "Can there be architecture without atmosphere?" the anthropologist Tim Ingold asks us (2016, 163).

> Can you imagine a building without the air that floods its volumes and circulates in its rooms, […] without the light that — at different times of day — illuminates certain surfaces while leaving others in shadow, and without the sounds of its inhabitants […]? Can you imagine a building that emits no scent, evokes no mood and harbours no feeling […]? Strange as it may seem, the history of architecture has largely been written as if its atmospheric component could be disregarded. (Ingold 2016, 163)

These days, a theory of atmospheres tout court is taking shape, borne out by the consolidation of an aesthetics and a phenomenology of atmospheres.[9] Academic interest has been kindled: or rather is ablaze. The nucleus of enquiry concerns first and foremost spatial perception, with claims that it is being examined from new points of view and with innovative methods. Innumerable disciplinary fields are taking part in an impressive expansion of the studies on spatial dynamics, driven by the energy of the so-called *spatial turn* (Griffero 2020d). This book attempts to shake up the supremacy of the (neo)phenomenological analysis of atmosphere, combining it with an experimental reading, sustained by insights provided from various scientific disciplines that explore the mechanisms of perception and behaviour of human beings (among them neuroscience). The (neo)phenomenological path of interpretation of subjective experiences inevitably constitutes the basis that triggers reflection, since the emotional sphere — which is the main

---

9   For an accurate and genuinely substantial "atmospheric bibliography" see (besides Griffero 2014a) the authoritative work promoted by *Atmospheric Spaces*, international community of research on the phenomenological-aesthetic dimension of atmospheric experience, coordinated by Tonino Griffero. The bibliographic review can be consulted online at www.atmosphericspaces.wordpress.com. It is a work in a continual state of updating, which takes the conventional start date of 1968 — the year in which the German psychiatrist Hubertus Tellenbach published his first book dedicated to the concept of atmosphere: *Geschmack und Atmosphäre* ("Taste and Atmosphere").

concern of those involved in architectural quality — "is not identifiable," in the first instance, "with physiological and neurobiological processes, if for nothing else because we don't live the emotions that assail us as neural processes at all" (Griffero 2005b, 12). As architecture professionals, scholars, and enthusiasts, so far we have relied on methods of enquiry directed at "a microgranularity and qualitative subjectivity frankly elusive in a naturalistic perspective (in third-person)" (Griffero, 12).

Without doubt, phenomenological research (at this point centred on the mutual influence wielded *from* and *on* architectonic places) provides a valid support, above all for the purpose of cutting loose from the primacy of psychic introspection when deciphering the relationship between perceiving individual and lived spatial experience. This interpretation of spatial perception goes beyond the dogma of the prioritized autonomy of the inner universe over external impulses and opens up to new manners of reflection. Greater attention on atmospheres sustains and promotes a global revision of the space-subjectivity connection, which implies "a critical stance on erecting rigid conceptual boundaries between emotion and affect, subject and object, nature and culture" (Bille, Bjerregaard, and Sørensen 2015, 33 citing Pile 2010). Among the authors who have begun to research a possible hybridization of principles between architectural poetics and (neuro)scientific knowledge, Robert Condia, designer and professor at Kansas State University,[10] stresses how "it is instructive that when perceiving architectural space, scientists and architects converge in a phenomenological, multi-sensory hypothesis" (Condia and Luczak 2014, 24).

Underlying this shift of horizon in critical-exegetic expectations, a certain level of dissatisfaction is also discernible, emergent from the nineties, vis-à-vis the models then available and predominant in the investigation and structure of material reality. We are today challenging those analytical approaches born of the so-called *cultural turn*, which in the last third of the twentieth century won over all the humanities and social disciplines (including the architecture department), giving priority to the observation of the impact of cultural factors, as expressed by language, social identity, and symbolic forms. In the contemporary era, there is the necessity to discuss

---

10   Among Robert Condia's main contributions to the interaction between architecture and neuroscience, with particular reference to those centred on the study of the biological bases of the aesthetic experience and the atmospheric dynamics, are both publications of a critical-theoretical nature (Condia 2020a, 2020b) and experimental design hypotheses (Rooney, Condia, and Loschky 2017).

a new renegotiation — conceptual and methodological — with regard to the study of the reality, which is currently undergoing an unprecedented wave of changes and technological progress. It is in this context that there emerges a reminder of materialist traditions, already scrutinised in previous years, which gives voice to a *new materialism*, increasingly reinforced by confirmations obtained from experimental applications, which legitimate the urgency for its consolidation (Coole and Frost 2010). On the momentum of this reversal of direction, we see a "rehabilitation of Baumgarten's idea of 'aesthetics' as 'theory of perceptible knowledge' — hence, distinct from a mere philosophy of art" (Oliva 2015, 228). At the same time, the theory of atmospheres, "felt in the first-person by the subject and originating from the qualities of the object, [...] prior to the division between the two poles of subjectivity and objectivity," lends itself to bringing into focus "the more elusive and enigmatic aspects of the human experience" (Oliva, 228). In conclusion, the growing importance of the atmospheric issue in this particular historical moment is not random, but mirrors — and at the same time provides unifying force to — the mutations that are taking place in the cultural milieu of the modern world as well as its scientific apparatus.

3. *In Praise of Atmospheres*

The unstoppable process of the aestheticism of reality, which — above all in advanced capitalist systems — overwhelms contemporary society (Edensor and Sumartojo 2015; Böhme 2017a), conferring to it the character of incessant *performance*, of perennial "mise-en-scène" (Böhme 2001) profusely charged with emotional appeal, has raised the atmospheric event to chief *catalyst of the aesthetic experience*. We aspire to an ideal of experience that quivers to be dynamic, global, immersive, and gratified not only from visual input. Today aesthetic judgement is increasingly understood as αἴσθησῐς (*aisthēsis*), or as the primitive meaning of sensitivity, as a form of knowledge of reality that passes through the body and the emotional nature of the individual, intrinsically rooted in their sensory and perceptual mechanisms. As Gernot Böhme clarifies "the aesthetics of atmospheres shifts attention away from the 'what' something represents, to the 'how' something is present" (1998, 114). "In this way," he goes on, "sensory perception as opposed to judgment is rehabilitated in aesthetics and the term 'aesthetic' is restored to its original meaning, namely the theory of perception" (Böhme, 114). The body, constituent foundation of every perceptive deviation, becomes the communicative threshold for intersubjective relationships and spatial interaction. Aided by the technological progress that has fired up the twentieth century, interest in the body has emerged increasingly potent, as never before. "Humans have had their bodies returned to them precisely by technological developments," highlights Gernot Böhme. "Released from being a labour force, the body potentially becomes the container of personal fulfilment" (2017b, 82).

On the other hand, a state of crisis is afflicting contemporary experiential activity: we are witnessing the progressive and continuous weakness of the corporeal dimension, affected by a process of dematerialisation — hyperstimulated — of references and contacts with the physical environment. The atmospheric approach claims a deeply felt urgency of presence, of integration between the individual and their architectonic surroundings. Professor Hans Ulrich Gumbrecht also exposes this tendency.

> The yearning for *Stimmung* has grown, because many of us — perhaps older people, above all — suffer from existence in an everyday world that often fails to surround and envelop us physically. Yearning for atmosphere and mood is a yearning for presence. (Gumbrecht 2012, 20)

The current cycle of dematerialisation has been triggered by the appearance — in the field of architectural and urban design — of *new perceptual-experiential frontiers*, which have assumed multiple forms: 1. — improved digital and automated building technologies, able to interact with the occupant even at a distance, communicating through sensors so accurately integrated in the body of the building as to be imperceptible but extremely conditioning; 2. — top quality materials, specifically designed to harmonize changes of state or temporarily alter form, colour, transparency, and density, in response to precise external stimuli (for example, if exposed to thermal, optical, or electrical stress); 3. — high-performance interfaces that allow work with the virtual, non-visible, and formless, that is with different spatial configurations than those habitually inherited from the past; 4. — the increase and tangling of the mass of flows, as much of information (one thinks of *big data* engulfed in complex algorithms) as people and things, which every architectural event is required to manage and coordinate; 5. — and new media, the sophisticated evolution of electronic devices that have accompanied the twentieth century. These have prompted powerful disorientation in sensory balance mechanisms, changing the ways in which today's human beings perceive and feel the space around them. "The effects of technology do not occur at the level of opinions or concepts, but alter sense ratios or patterns of perception steadily and without any resistance," affirms the Canadian sociologist Marshall McLuhan, back in the sixties (1964, 33). "As an extension and expediter of the sense life, any medium at once affects the entire field of the senses" (McLuhan, 54). The relative repercussions on our perceptual-environmental plasticity are obvious today. The emergence of new digital and immersive spatial domains, the insistent push towards virtual interaction between animate and inanimate bodies, the widespread diffusion of internet on individual devices as well as the aggravation of personal isolation (also in terms of occupation of the physical space, both public and private) determine a profound shift of sensory paradigms, through the dispersion of impulses and dilation of emotional contagion. The sphere of feeling is torn and dematerialises, developing unusual forms of perception and experience — blurring into the *third element*, as Peter Sloterdijk (2014, 137) calls it, the territory of atmospheric sensibility.

The atmospheric approach may be an effective response to the ongoing changes, stirred up by the current of "media-emotional manipulation" that "the aesthetisation of politics and social life in the late-capitalistic 'scenic' economy results in" (Griffero 2014a, 7). Furthermore, such an approach seems to face the underway process of fragmentation of contemporary society, in which individuals are increasingly concentrated on themselves, closed in their own emotional microcosm, detached from spatial ideals of collective sharing. People tenaciously try to obtain their own bubble in which to find some sort of emotional stability, also aided by digital technologies that produce a "redistribution of sensory connections" (De Freitas and Rousell 2021, 227). Atmospheric space satisfies this need for intensified intimacy, in that it is the space of our physical presence, the space we perceive with our body, the space that includes us. Today, architecture cannot be limited to designing static and defined spaces, it is above all required to suggest *spatial experiences* that are as multifocal and heterarchical as possible, provided with the sensory malleability capable of resonating with innumerable different subjects. This is why we are encountering "the elevation of the atmospheric to theory-worthiness" and now "one would have to speak of a discovery of the indeterminate that has enabled — perhaps for the first time in the history of thought — [...] the formless to join the domain of theory-capable realities" (Sloterdijk 2016, 34–35).

V
To Perceive the Invisible

1. *Experiencing Architecture*

After sifting through the ample range of interpretations, gleaned from and fine-tuned by the panorama of the architectural culture,[1] the needle of the compass has come to rest on the pole registering atmospheric phenomenon as *perceptive experience*. The aim is to attempt to set up an architectural theory of atmosphere of an experiential nature,[2] inspired by notions of a biological matrix.

A premise is imperative: lived experience is recognised as having the primacy of knowing how to confer meaning to architectural existence (von Meiss 1990; Johnson 2015; Plummer 2016). A principle that is well expressed in the words of the Scottish psychiatrist Ronald David Laing: "the physical environment unremittingly offers us possibilities of experience, or curtails them. The fundamental human significance of architecture stems from this" (1967, 28). The experiential vocation of architecture is manifested — above all — through its atmospheres (Sumartojo and Pink 2019). Crystallizing itself as a full and complete experience of the architectural substance, here atmosphere is deciphered as *the condition of emotional resonance and subsequent consonance between the perceiving subject and their architectonically arranged surroundings*.[3]

---

1 See chapter III "Atlas of Atmospheres."
2 Sturdier theoretical foundations are required. The study of the atmospheric effects on consumer behaviour, for example, is one of the most long-running fields (Kotler 1973) where an experimental approach has been adopted. Despite the accumulated evidence, "there is a strong need for additional theory development in this area" to prevent "atheoretical descriptions of effects" (Turley and Milliman 2000, 208).
3 Consonance but also its opposite, dissonance. "We are traversed by [...] consonances and dissonances with the external world with no more justification than the 'mood' of the moment — to which the environment and architecture

Thus, what occurs is that by means of its inherent spatial charge, the architectural action transmits to the physical surroundings an emotional potential, modelling a perceptive, stratified and multi-sensory, atmospheric state in which the individual — spatially immersed — would be able to interiorise and simulate certain architectural properties. It is assumed that the atmosphere contributes to initiating and defining a relationship of empathic symbiosis between the animate body (the sentient individual — equipped with senses and sensibility) and a collection of inanimate objects (forming the intentionally designed choreography of architectural elements that populate and characterise their surroundings). Or, again, in other words, it is supposed that atmosphere can become the *medium of empathic perception of the field of stimuli and energies staged by the architectural presence*.

As Tonino Griffero clarifies, "perception gathers the overall sensible-emotional atmosphere of an object or place before any sort of analytical scrutiny (conceptual and objectual)" (2005a, 301). Borrowing an expression that Silvia Benedito synthesized to introduce the theme of atmosphere in a design seminar at Harvard Graduate School of Design (GSD), one can say that "atmospheres are the immediate perception of the invisible (that get revealed) and the actual relation to our own *natureness*" (2013, 2: original italics).

The comparison with (neuro)biological[4] extraction theories, derived from a previously metabolised transition of the phenomenological and aesthetics repertoire, takes part not to further emphasize the conceptual and cerebral component of the experiential dynamics, but to valorise the centrality of the body in perceiving the architectural substance (Robinson 2011; Tidwell 2013, 2015). The assumption is that "an atmosphere is not simply a space but a combination of space and activity — something produced by the people within the space" (Thibaud 2014b, 71). Atmosphere comes from the immersive and integral contact of the individual with the architectonic

---

    contribute in a fundamental way" (Pérez-Gómez 2016, 90). Being part of the co-production of the atmospheric event and perceiving its emotional content does not imply becoming affectively attuned to it. Individuals can feel in tune with a specific atmosphere, but they can also remain insensitive or reject it. There is a distinction between *sensing the presence* of an atmosphere and *being actually involved* by it (cf. De Matteis et al. 2019, § 40–42).

4   The added value that recent discoveries in biology, psychology, and neuroscience can bring to the aesthetic-architectural debate (and to the dialogue with human sciences more in general) is manifold. See Di Dio and Gallese 2009; Chatterjee and Vartanian 2014; Gallese 2019; Mallgrave and Gepshtein 2021.

context; it activates and promotes interaction of the subject's multiple manners of spatial perception, shaking up their emotional sphere and influencing their cognitive faculties. "Whatever we know about reality," explains the psychologist Ulrich Neisser, pioneer of the cognitive approach,[5] "has been mediated not only by the organs of sense but by complex systems which interpret and reinterpret sensory information." "The term 'cognition,'" continues Neisser, "refers to all the processes by which the sensory input is transformed, reduced, elaborated, stored, recovered" (1967 as cited in Kandel et al. 2013, 371).

There is a two-way influence in the exchange of impulses and reactions between the body and its surroundings. Somatosensory information detected along sensitive exteroceptive (skin) and proprioceptive (muscles) routes links up with information recorded in peripersonal and extrapersonal spaces[6] (among which visual, olfactory, and acoustic stimuli). Perception of the external spatial contingencies emerges from the activation of emotional and motor skills, archived in the memory, and from mental representations modifiable with experience. The human being is a complex "biological, psychological, socio-political being" (Kiesler 1949, 738), which designers find hard to comprehend; it is a unique creature — synthetic unity of form and matter, genetically determined but at the same time moulded by the environment in which it has grown. As Richard Neutra recalls, "neither physically nor biochemically nor sociologically can the individual really be segregated or isolated as a separate entity" (1954, 12).

> Through the process of respiration the organism is chemically so united with its environment that the two can be separated only in the abstract way in which we separate the water of two tributaries which have flowed together into a common river bed. Organisms are immersed to fusion in their chemical as well as their social setting; *they literally live on and in one another.* (Neutra 1954, 12: original italics)

---

5   With the expression *cognitive psychology*, we mean a series of researches and theories relative to the study of human behaviour, based on mental processes (and hence not observable) that connect stimulus to response.
6   "The brain constructs multiple representations of space," reveal recent neuroscientific researches. "A key division is between near, peripersonal space and far, extrapersonal space representations. [...] Peripersonal space defines the region of space immediately surrounding our bodies in which objects can be grasped and manipulated. By contrast, extrapersonal space refers to the space which is crucial for the control of somatic, head and arm movements" (Di Pellegrino and Làdavas 2015, 126).

This leads to my hypothesis that the body can establish an empathic relationship with the surrounding architectonic setting, inwardly simulating certain attributes (such as shape, size, colours, and materiality).[7] This experience would allow the individual a contextual understanding of their surroundings, which is immediate and preconscious — as well as interactive, and deeply suggested by the emotional impressions afforded by atmospheric tension. Within this research scenario, the presupposed dynamic of (emotional and corporeal) empathy is analysed through the interpretative filter of the *embodied simulation*,[8] an experimental perspective, recently put forward, which assimilates the simulative theories defined by the cognitive social approach, integrating them with the study of neurophysiological mechanisms of mirroring in actions, emotions, and bodily sensations. The presumed neural correlate of this functional process is the system of *mirror neurons*.[9] These prove to be capable of translating the sensory qualities of an observed object, or of a recognised action, in a motor programme of interaction.

> Every action, whatever it may be — from turning your eyes to look over this page and pick up the cup of tea that accompanies reading — is characterised by the presence of an aim. Even *movements*, for example flexing the fingers of your hand, can be carried out for different purposes (to pick up a glass, scratch your head, simply fidget with your fingers, etc.). The presence of different aims makes different *actions* of these same movements. (Gallese 2006, 300: original italics)

Mirror neurons don't decode a movement, but an action, understood as the association of "movement + aim," and they facilitate comprehension of its meaning; which is to say, they can play an important role in the recognition of the intentional inclination of the observed action. Expressing the concept of intersubjectivity as intercorporeality[10] and extending these theoretical horizons to the dominion of spatial dynamics (and, consequently, to the

---

7 Or rather, the so-called *generators of atmosphere* (for more, see the section of the present chapter entitled "first property: atmosphere is composite"). See also Böhme 2001, 2013b, 2017b; Zumthor 2006; Edensor and Sumartojo 2015; Schönhammer 2018; Canepa et al. 2019; Martin, Nettleton, and Buse 2019.
8 See Gallese 2005; Freedberg and Gallese 2007; Gallese and Sinigaglia 2011.
9 See Rizzolatti and Sinigaglia 2008.
10 "The discovery of mirror neurons gives us a new empirically founded notion of intersubjectivity first and foremost conceived as intercorporeality — the mutual resonance of intentionally meaningful sensorimotor behaviors. [...] In many situations, we can directly grasp the meaning of other people's basic actions thanks to the motor equivalence between what others do and what we can do" (Gallese 2017a, 44).

sensorimotor relations that they express),[11] it is plausible and interesting to suppose that every architectural landscape, through its atmospheric epiphanies, enters into resonance with the subpersonal components[12] of the individual and is interiorised as subjective experience. To establish a relationship (even just a visual one) with a place, a room, or certain architectural details, would imply, therefore, unconsciously "simulating" the motor actions, emotions, and corporeal sensations that "those spaces and objects evoke" (Gallese 2015, XIII). And this would occur through triggered atmospheric transport. "Atmospheres then seem to be bridge-qualities, founded on a corporeal communication without any real contact between user and object," clarifies Tonino Griffero. "Their suggestions are perceivable as virtual movements" (2014c, 16). The *atmospheric continuum* that the architectural scene sets up, understood as an ensemble of physical-environmental factors that produce (multi)sensory input, is thought to be capable of conditioning emotional states, moods, and behaviour in individuals who dynamically interact with it (Schreuder et al. 2016).

2. Paradigm Shift

Through the analysis of the atmospheric content of architectonic matter, the entire spectrum of expressive qualities of the constructed landscape is highlighted, with particular vividness, and not only the shapes revealed from the retinal scan. Today, there is a very strong need in architecture for renewed attention to *corporeality*, evaluated in its composite and multisensory essence.[13] Atmospheric outburst requires the involvement of the whole body, or better, of the indivisible body-brain-mind system, in which the individual is identified and observed in their interaction with the external environment. The body is the epicentre of our faculties of perception and appreciation of the sensible beauty of the architectural

---

11 Every sensorimotor relationship with external physical reality is connected as much to emotional and affective aspects as to mechanisms of mirroring and motor simulation. "When we observe three-dimensional objects," explains Professor Gallese, "we simulate the actions that such objects invite us to carry out" (2015, XIII). Over the years, Vittorio Gallese became one of the protagonists of research into mirror neurons, in that he is the member of the team at the University of Parma, coordinated by Giacomo Rizzolatti (responsible for this important discovery at the beginning of the nineties), that is most focused on the reflection of potential consequences that mirroring processes have on an aesthetic-philosophical level.
12 That is, at a nonconscious and preconscious level.
13 See the section in this chapter entitled "third property: atmosphere is multisensory."

organism; it is the vector that allows us to breathe the pervading atmosphere; it is the horizon of manifestation of our emotions. Robert Condia teaches us that "the body is the measure of architecture and the most important tool of the architect" (2021, 3).[14]

Traditionally, architects have approached the atmospheric resource with a certain lack of awareness, or rather they have let themselves be inspired by their intuition. "The most essential architectural qualities seem to arise instinctively from the designer's sense of his/her body rather than conscious and intellectually identified objectives" (Pallasmaa 2013, 53). According to Juhani Pallasmaa, this principle would justify the atmospheric attitude of some architects, such as Frank Lloyd Wright, Alvar Aalto, and Sigurd Lewerentz, who "have expressed an understanding, or at least an appreciation, of atmospheres in their writing" (2014c, 68). To date, atmospheric production has been interpreted as the spontaneous conclusion of those design processes, originated as existential explorations, in which the architect's professional expertise merges with their life experiences, projections of their private imagination as well as the knowledge of their body[15] — that is, every nuance of their person.

As Gernot Böhme suggests (2013b), taking up the early twentieth century reflections of August Endell ([1908] 2018), an inversion of terms of reference within the design paradigm is to be hoped: the focus should move from the static body of the building to the living body of the individual, from the design of edifices to that of *spaces*, promoting subjective introspection instead of merely technical-objective inquiries. Or, better still, the "necessary paradigm shift," as Silvia Benedito launches the challenge, requires conceiving "space as atmosphere" (2021, 17). Iconic and sensationalist architecture, that is spreading in today's society, is asked to contend with a design approach that is more sensitive to the history of the individual, concentrating on their biological roots, to satisfy human

---

14 "The body's instrumental function is etymologically indicated in words like 'organism' and 'organ,' which derive from the Greek word *organon*, meaning 'tool'" (Shusterman 2006, 9).
15 To improve the instrumental use of the body, the American philosopher Richard Shusterman (1999, 2000, 2006) recommends three steps: 1. — an *analytic* preparation to understand the nature of somatic perceptions; 2. — a *pragmatic* study of previously proposed methodologies to enhance the body's experience and utilization; 3. — a *practical* training based on physical exercise.

needs instead of frustrating them.[16] Such is the scene of contemporary architecture, scrutinized by a critical eye:

> In our time, architecture is threatened by two opposite processes: instrumentalisation and aestheticisation. On the one hand, our secular, materialist and quasi-rational culture is turning buildings into mere instrumental structures, devoid of mental meaning, for the purposes of utility and economy. On the other hand, in order to draw attention and facilitate instant seduction, architecture is increasingly turning into the fabrication of seductively aestheticised images without roots in our existential experience and devoid of authentic desire of life. (Pallasmaa 2011b, 119)

3. Scientific Grounding

Acknowledging the fundamental role carried out by our emotions and simulative-mimetic skills to interact with architectonically structured space, one can presume that human beings already elaborate perceived atmospheric stimuli at a neurophysiological level.[17] Thus the decision to explore the atmospheric phenomenon, as mentioned above, from an experimental perspective of a biological origin,[18] with which to weigh the supposed importance that the phenotypical ties occupy in the creative and perceptive act of atmospheres.[19] The primary intent is to evaluate the existence of an — eventual — (neuro)biological basis of the atmospheric sense, appointed to valorise the physiological origin of our spatial interactions. One wonders, that is, if architectural atmosphere,

---

16 Nowadays, the material and psychological necessities that an architect must satisfy to gratify the future occupant's well-being, at the point in which they intervene on their environment, controlling and transforming it, are increasingly complex and amply advanced with respect to the basic request of shelter fulfilled by the primitive hut.

17 The focus of the analysis shifts to the nervous system (central and peripheral), of which activities and functioning mechanisms are studied.

18 Albeit, inevitably, reinforced by suggestions of phenomenological and aesthetics influence.

19 The naturalization of the atmospheric experience, adopting an approach of a (neuro) scientific type, allows a change in perspective from which to observe and consider the weight that biological, environmental, and cultural factors have in shaping the experience. The modern human being is, in terms of biological structures, the same as thousands of years ago. A study of the neurological dimension leads one to ask if "through these newly developing [experimental] insights we may expect to determine true physiological constants" (1954, 182) — a question on which (with very current lucidity) Richard Neutra reflected back in the fifties.

socio-cultural construct par excellence,[20] also has its *neurophysiological correlate*, scientifically determinable and measurable, and able to integrate the poetic-personal dimension.

The element of conjunction, which is the intermediary between the scientific doctrine and theoretical architectural speculation, is the *body*. A strategy per se that is not at all new. "In the past, many architectural theorists already speculated about the body-architecture relationship," but it was done "usually in formal theories lacking any experiential or perceptual bases" (Papale et al. 2016, 2). Among the different experiences, we can cite the following directions of investigation, many of which are today living an intense season of revival, thanks to the advance of research supported by scientific evidence criteria: 1. — principles of proportional harmony, established on geometric analogies, correspondence of symmetry, and mathematical correlations;[21] 2. — the model of biophilia, the scientific hypothesis that identifies, in human beings, innate attraction towards nature and vital processes; 3. — experimental approaches to research of spatial dynamics influenced by today's embedded, embodied, enactive, extended, and affective theories of cognition (the 4EA cognition paradigm);[22] 4. — study of the emotional impact of visual stimuli, in the light that the fruition and design of architecture are broadly based on visual input;[23] 5. — the multisensory reinterpretation of the architectural process, in open opposition to the concept of ocularcentric architecture, criticised for the excessive emphasis that is reserved for vision, as primary source of aesthetic appreciation (Pallasmaa 1998, 2012a; Robinson 2012).

---

20 Of extremely composite content, of which the *Atlas of Atmospheres* outlined the first map (see chapter III).
21 Over all, the module of the golden section has exercised a very strong fascination over the centuries.
22 For a detailed study of *4E approach to cognition*, see Newen, De Bruin, and Gallagher 2018; Carney 2020. Regarding the current *4EA cognitive science and philosophy*, see Ward and Stapleton 2012. Sarah Robinson (2022) suggests practical strategies aimed to integrate principles of 4E cognition into architectural design education.
23 Many studies demonstrated visual dominance over other sensory modalities in spatial perception, a dominance that is also socially and culturally reinforced (Hutmacher 2019).

This is where the search for the biological roots of the atmospheric phenomenon comes in. Technological progress[24] and the new humanist models collaborate in finding empirical confirmation around the changes of corporeal state that it is supposed accompany the emotional responsiveness solicited by atmosphere. With the aim of evaluating and mapping the biological correlates, innovative experimental protocols[25] are being drawn, with which physiological parameters of the body are measured[26] and neural activity of the brain monitored, turning to techniques of neurophysiology or neuroimaging.[27] In parallel, the psychological components are analysed, using self-assessment tools,[28] which gather descriptions of the lived experience as consciously perceived by the individual under examination.[29]

24 To be very brief, we can say that neuroscience is a hybrid domain studying the brain, or, more generally, the nervous system. Enlarging the field of focus, we realise that the goal of neuroscience is "to understand the biological mechanisms that account for mental activity." It seeks "to understand the biological underpinnings of our emotional life" (Albright et al. 2000, s1). In the second half of the twentieth century, the neuroscientific discipline is overwhelmed by a phase of intense and rapid growth, which has lasted up to the present day. It accelerates from year to year, so much so that the contemporary era is facing the stunning effects of a heavy intoxication of "neuromania" (Legrenzi and Umiltà 2011), which exploded in the recent past with its promises and progressively consolidated results, but also with the weight of its limits (Fitzgerald and Callard 2014). Many factors have contributed to this propulsion. Above all else, the improvement of neurophysiological and neuroimaging techniques. Their potential is revolutionary. These tools allow us to carry out *in vivo* surveys on human subjects, studying them in their normal behaviour or in conditions affected by pathology. We are talking of highly specialised and precise methods, intended for instantaneous and direct observation of the brain's superior functions. Regardless of the chosen technology, the act of monitoring cerebral activity is never an invasive operation, much less painful. Before, not having such equipment available, there were basically three possibilities: 1. — to work on neurological patients affected by cerebral lesions and therefore suffering a deficit of cognitive functioning; 2. — to carry out post-mortems; 3. — to experiment with therapeutic hypotheses during neurosurgical operations and gather the "unexpected consequences" (Gabrieli, Ghosh, and Whitfield-Gabrieli 2015, 11).
25 See, for example, the research project RESONANCES (2021–2024), funded by the European Union's Horizon 2020 research and innovation programme under the Marie Skłodowska-Curie grant agreement no. 101025132 (www.resonances-project.com).
26 Such as the respiratory rate, heartbeats, blood pressure, and skin temperature.
27 See Bell et al. 2018; Bower, Tucker, and Enticott 2019; Mostafavi 2021.
28 Viz. written or oral accounts (such as questionnaires, interviews, and audio/video recordings), but also non-verbal exercises (such as drawings, picture-oriented rating diagrams, body maps, and photographs).
29 Methods that, although not registering automatic and instinctive reactions, but subjective interpretations (regulated in a reflexive way and usually lexically

The structuring of the atmospheric event on (neuro)biologically plausible bases, as a *state of resonance and consonance (sensorimotor, emotive, and cognitive) between the perceiving subject and their architectonically arranged environment*, has led to the composition of an anthology of scientific theories, expressly selected and formalised in an organic research hypothesis. In synthesis, four key elements support this reading: 1. — the multisensory nature of perceptual processes; 2. — the dynamics of embodiment, that highlights the indispensable role of the corporeal presence and the body-brain-mind unit entrenched in its environmental context; 3. — the emotional content of the spatial experience; 4 — the phenomenon of emotional and physiological empathy.

4. *The Polyphony of the Senses*

In summary, atmosphere is a *spatial concept*, it is the "primary and, to a certain degree, basic object of perception" (Böhme 1991, 34), tied to the combination of the qualitative traits of a certain physical domain and of the corporeal sensitivity of the individual immersed in it. Both poles of the perception circuit are necessary. "Despite our modern, often-egotistical self-understanding, we cannot have emotions without the external prompts of the environment" (Pérez-Gómez 2016, 24). We incessantly build our personal atmosphere, an intimate cocoon of "bilateral perception that has nothing metaphorical about it" (Griffero 2014a, 118). *Atmosphere is a state of resonance with reality mediated by architecture.* And, in making the expressive qualities of the space echo, atmospheric perception — or perhaps it would be more correct to speak of *co-perception* (Griffero 2014a) — becomes an experience of *sensory synthesis*, connoted by specific constituent properties: 1. — atmosphere is *composite*, that is a cohesive force that orchestrates multiple factors (the so-called "generators of atmosphere"); 2. — atmosphere is *unfocused*, since it is primarily assimilated thanks to peripheral and nonconscious perceptual mechanisms; 3. — atmosphere is *multisensory*; 4. — atmosphere is *multimodal*, or rather it manages and integrates the ambient stimuli independently of the sensory modality in which the raw data are acquired; 5. — atmosphere is *kinaesthetic* and *haptic*: it transcends the filter of vision; 6. — lastly,

---

expressed), provide an important element of reference with which to compare the recorded (neuro)physiological data, since they have been widely tested and submitted to rigid validation processes. "Describing how emotion experiences are caused does not substitute for a description of what is felt" (Barrett et al. 2007, 374).

atmosphere is *instinctive*, capable of triggering itself autonomously with respect to the cognitive mediation of the individual living it.

First property: atmosphere is composite

The composite complexity in which an architectonic space is organized is — first of all — grasped in its entirety, before being analysed in each part and detail. This is the teaching provided by neuroscience.

> In vision, as in other cognitive operations, various features — motion, depth, form, and color — occur together in a unified percept. This unity is achieved not by one hierarchical neural system but by multiple areas in the brain that are fed by parallel but interacting neural pathways. (Kandel et al. 2021, 499)

Reality, although being x-rayed point by point, is not recorded as a cloud of signs; it is clotted in a unitary and interactive association of its components, which should not be considered as a mere additive synthesis of single elementary sensations. The idea of an all-embracing, rather than a fragmentary, perception was scientifically formulated for the first time at the beginning of the twentieth century, by the exponents of the Gestalt School (Albright et al. 2000).[30] Thanks to a concatenation of reciprocal relationships between elements, the perception we have of a complex scene is different from that relative to the single parts that make it up. Richard Neutra uses the metaphor of mastication to describe this mechanism.

> In our everyday life we are assailed continuously by a chaotic complexity of forms, shades, colors, smells, noises. But a differentiating, abstracting, and then synthesizing process takes place, until the chaos around us is somehow articulated into more or less distinct objects and organized entities. This mastication of an outer world in individual bites, followed by a suffusing of all particles into a digestible world picture, is a device not unlike chewing, salivation, and digestion for the assimilation of physical food. (Neutra 1954, 123)

---

30 As we read in Kandel, neuroscience textbook par excellence, which, evolving from edition to edition, has become a sacred text for generations of medical students, "more recent psychophysical and neurophysiological work has lent further support to [several] principles" formulated by the psychologists of the Gestalt (Kandel et al. 2013, 494).

Upheld by the theoretical evidence provided by the neuroscientist Michael Arbib, in connection with the fact that perception and comprehension of reality set out from the complex entity to then disassociate and shift onto its details, Juhani Pallasmaa affirms that in the same way atmospheric perception "is an immediate experience of the whole, the entity, and only later can one distinguish the details that are part of it" (interviewed in Havik and Tielens 2013b, 37). Atmosphere, in so far as it is a total experience, is the result of an indeterminate interaction of *generators of atmosphere*,[31] which may be found both in macroscopically perceptible characteristics and in the qualities of a psychological order, which are less intelligible.

Architecture and design have focused overly on the creation of things, without acquiring an explicit awareness of the fact that architectural and design elements are *generators*, to wit, they must radiate something and contribute to the production of atmospheres. (Böhme 2001, 178: original italics)

In the architectural field, generators of atmosphere "are above all the geometric structures and corporeal constellations" that are designed (Böhme 2017b, 93). They can be as much "of an objective kind" (such as movement suggestions afforded by the shape and geometry of the architectonic body) as "non-objective or non-physical," such as light and sound (Böhme, 92). In his book *Aisthetik* (2001), Gernot Böhme analyses the potential relationships that exist between the atmosphere generating elements and the attributes of the atmospheres themselves. The latter were initially[32] subdivided into five classes of *atmospheric characters* (101–104), where by "character" we mean the essence of the atmospheres, or "the characteristic manner in which they impress" (87). The characters regularly overlap, but one can always make out one that is preponderant: 1. — *synaesthetic reverberations*, produced by specific sensory data (such as colours, sounds, smells, and noises) that transpire from the architectonic materiality through their sensible effects and are initially perceived in aggregate; 2. — *movement impressions* (that is, kinaesthetic suggestions such as sensations of volume, load,

---

31 "The making of atmospheres is restricted to the arrangement of the conditions under which an atmosphere can appear. These conditions I call *generators*" (Böhme 2017b, 161: original italics). See also note 7 of this chapter.

32 More recently, as in the essay "The Presence of Living Bodies in Space" (collected in Böhme 2017b, 81–95), three groups of characters are highlighted in particular: *synaesthetic reverberations, movement impressions,* and *social characters*. See also Böhme 2013b.

and density, which can render a space oppressive, solemn, vast, or poignant), transmitted through the design of shapes and masses; 3. — *social characters* (such as the sense of power, wealth, or elegance), put across by means of symbols and signs, of culturally significant content, which compete to contextualise the social condition or historical era to which there is a desire to associate a given environment, embedding well recognisable conventional canons;[33] 4. — *dispositions of mind* (that is the characters comparable to the mood tendency induced thanks to a specific atmosphere), evoked by the scenic charge, for example, of a theatre set or landscape views of gardens and belvederes; 5. — *communicative characters* (capable of connoting the tone of a communicative situation, which might be friendly, taut, aggressive, or depressed), expressed by gestures, mimicry, the timbre of the voice, and the physiognomy of the person occupying a space.

Gernot Böhme's research leads to a formalised, systematic, and elastically precise cataloguing, very remote from the attempts at diagnosis of the atmospheric substance put forward by architects, interested above all in compiling vague biographical inventories of their own design approach. Of course, the most famous architecturally formulated atmospheric index is that compiled by Peter Zumthor. His recipe discloses a concatenation of reflections (twelve elements, to be exact), which — by his own admission — are "highly personal" considerations, nothing more than "products of sensitivities" (2006, 21): 1. — the "body of architecture," or the concrete presence of a building: its structure, mass, and surfaces; 2. — the "materials compatibility," resulting from their natural composition, origin, visual impact, the various possibilities of reciprocal reaction to a particular critical closeness and the relative illusion of lightness that they might transmit; 3. — the "sound of a space," shaped on the configuration of surfaces, the reflective and cushioning properties of the materials adopted, the friction of the air on bodies, the wind, as well as the echoes of memories emerging from the past and the sense of familiarity;[34] 4. — the "temperature of a space," which harmonises with the physical and psychological temperature of its occupants; 5. — the "surrounding objects," tied to the real life of the building and of the people living

---

33 Imagine, just to cite an example, the "petit-bourgeois" atmosphere of an apartment.
34 "There are buildings that have wonderful sounds, telling me I can feel at home, I'm not alone. I suppose I just can't get rid of that image of my mother, and actually I don't want to" (Zumthor 2006, 33).

there, enabling them to feel at home, at their ease; 6. — the equilibrium "between composure and seduction," regulated by the motor impulses that shapes and objects in the space can stimulate, relaxing or inviting movement;[35] 7. — the "tension between interior and exterior," communicated by signs, thresholds, passages, breaks between public and private, between seen and hidden, between vanity and reserve; 8. — the "levels of intimacy," a delicate balance of proportions, geometries, distances, masses, volumes, and voids tailored to human scale;[36] 9. — the "light on things," which brings out their beauty, when it manages to add value to the characteristics of the materials as well as when it produces fluctuations of luminosity and shade, which plot a rhythmic succession of stimuli; 10. (appendix one) — "architecture as surroundings," which becomes an integral part of people's lives, a loved place, manufacturer of memories;[37] 11. (appendix two) — the "coherence," namely coherence between the parts that make up the whole, the weave of relationships in tension between space, function, and form; 12. (appendix three) — the "beautiful form," which translates into the pure emotion that the body of architecture exudes, if the composition of each design choice satisfies the expectations of architect and inhabitant.

It is obvious that any list of this type only has the value of an indicative guide in exploring the atmospheric territory, but it is not plausible to transmute similar subjective intuitions into scientifically objective models, without due premises and simplifications. As Alberto Pérez-Gómez stresses, the difficulty is not in compiling a list like this (all told, a simple operation), but in understanding that "our embodied experience where meaning actually appears is always *primarily* synesthetic and enactive" (2016, 31: original italics). In other words, "it is never possible to simply add one characteristic to another as a factor in an equation" (Pérez-Gómez, 31–32).

---

[35] "Let me give you an example in connection with some thermal baths we built. It was incredibly important for us to induce a sense of freedom of movement, a milieu for strolling, a mood that had less to do with directing people than seducing them. Hospital corridors are all about directing people" (Zumthor 2006, 41).

[36] "It is interesting that there are things bigger than me that can intimidate me" (Zumthor 2006, 53).

[37] "It increases the pleasure of my work when I imagine a certain building being remembered by someone in twenty-five years' time. Perhaps because that was where he kissed his first girlfriend or whatever" (Zumthor 2006, 65).

Second property: atmosphere is unfocused

Returning to a suggestion of Juhani Pallasmaa,[38] who on several occasions confronted the theme of atmosphere with Peter Zumthor,[39] it is valid to hypothesize that "atmosphere is altogether an unfocused quality." "It has to be experienced in an unfocused and partly unconscious manner" (Havik and Tielens 2013b, 45). Namely, "peripheral perception is the perceptive mode through which we grasp atmospheres" (Pallasmaa 2014a, 244). This observation turns out to be exact, above all, regarding the analysis of visual information. The human eye operates two perfectly integrated procedures of vision: *central vision*, which polarises on given objects, details, and fragments of the scene, and is, for example, sensitive to colour; and *peripheral vision*, which seems to provide a primary structural representation, or a sort of overall picture. Any detail falling outside the fovea[40] (the central region of the retina where the vision is clearest in absolute) nourishes the peripheral sensibility, deputed to the detection of contours, contrasts, and movement.

Peripheral vision directs the progressive — and fundamental — process of selection of sensory information that crowds the visual field, that is, it performs the task of choosing the elements of interest to explore; an excessive input of data would weigh down the analysis of our surrounding space, slowing it and strewing it with lacuna. Thence, the operation of approximation of the complexity of the physical reality in the indistinct, out of focus, and atmospheric, is a physiologically necessary act. It happens that "as we look out on the world we focus on specific objects or scenes that have particular interest and exclude others" (Kandel et al. 2000,

---

38 Juhani Pallasmaa (b. 1936), today a necessary reference on atmospheric enquiry within the architectural community, has rigorously dedicated himself to the study of the atmospheric phenomenon from the beginning of the 2010s. Surprised by the vertiginous growth of interest that was gradually surrounding the atmospheric topic, he maintains that it follows the course of other tendencies of research, as "interests in the senses, in sensuality, in the idea of the narrative, and more recently, in the relationship between architecture and neuroscience" (Havik and Tielens 2013b, 35).
39 Both in a direct manner (Andersen 2012) and an indirect form (Böhme 2013d).
40 Our eyes can see clearly only a reduced portion of the space around us, which corresponds to the area defined by 1.5±2 degrees central to the visual field with respect to the axis of the fovea (the zone that possesses the maximum visual acuity). Therefore, the vision of the fovea touches and brings into focus only a hundred and eightieth of the space in which we are immersed.

401). The eye concentrates on what is reputed to be important. "Humans therefore constantly move their eyes so that scenes of interest are projected onto the fovea" (Kandel et al., 509). From here comes the sensation that we always see everything clearly. Peripheral vision is weak in human beings, anaesthetised with respect to other animal species. And yet it is essential since, when one enters into contact with any architectural experience, it is the visual recognition that prevails over all the sensory interaction activating with the spatial domain. Of late, some research, focused on the interpolation of architectural concepts with neuroscientific principles, have confronted the theme of the double visual filter, finding that the atmospheric dynamics is strongly mediated by the peripheral visual system.

> Given the visual mechanisms of vision from the retina to the dorsal and ventral streams, the experience of architecture simultaneously operates within the central and peripheral visual fields through focal and ambient modes of vision. Due to this fluid state, architecture stands as a unique type of environmental stimulus which can transition between object and scene perception along a cognitive spectrum of visual and attentive responses unlike most other stimuli. [...] There is an architecture which we intellectually assess through our focal attention and an architecture atmosphere we perceive through our phenomenal awareness of [the] surrounding environment. (Rooney 2016, 50)

Third property: atmosphere is multisensory

"Space as atmosphere is nothing but vibration or *pure conductivity*," declares the German philosopher Peter Sloterdijk (2014, 136: original italics). The swarm of conscious, semiconscious, and nonconscious sensations, diffused by the architectural surroundings, that sensorially stimulate the individual immersed within, produces a *continuous and integrated perceptive medium*. As such, it powers up various sensory channels simultaneously, even going so far as to elicit, at times, a "moment of trance" (Tanizaki [1933] 2001, 25). "Polyphony of the senses," was the name given to it by another philosopher, the Frenchman Gaston Bachelard (1971, 6). Human beings depend on their surroundings — also — to provide for their primary need for signals, as much of a biological nature (like sensory stimuli) as a social type (such as messages sent by facial expression and gesticulations from their fellows, those with whom they cohabit). Think of how we react to the void, the total absence of signals. "The blank often makes us shudder," notes Richard Neutra. "In general, [humans feel] prompted to fill a vacant space with pattern. Children are fairly impelled to scrawl on a blank wall" (1954, 103). The atmospheric tension draws to itself the combination of the percepts triggered by the architectural experience, operating a *function of stabilisation between diverse signals*; it harmonises the sensory stimulation exerted by the external world on the internal homeostasis,[41] which oversees all our activities, both somatic and mental.

In the coagulation into atmospheric sense, the environmental flows are not processed as a series of distinct and separate sensory reactions, they merge into an indissoluble amalgam of multiple and complementary interactions. Atmospheric sensibility gathers architectural experience in its multisensory essence, promoting a close reciprocal influence among the different senses[42] and a fusion of their informative content.[43] Firstly, it should be noted that the human organism is not only endowed with the five classical senses — of vision, hearing, touch, taste, and smell (Pallasmaa 2016b). There exist, for example, the somatic senses of pain, temperature, pruritus, and proprioception (controlling posture and body segments)[44]; and the vestibular sense of balance.

All sensory systems, when stimulated, react to four common elementary properties: mode, location, intensity, and duration of the stimulus. Each sensory system has evolved to respond to a specific type of energy present in the physical environment, which then is converted through its receptors into electrical signals. In particular, the visual system is activated by the light and through its photoreceptors elaborates the information relative to a distinct bandwidth of the electromagnetic spectrum; the hearing system is activated by a distinct bandwidth of vibratory energy in the air; the somatic sensations can react to energetic stimuli of a chemical, thermal, or mechanic nature; the systems of taste and smell are sensitive to narrow categories of chemical energy. In studying the principles of human perception, we have acquired a great deal more understanding with regard to the sensory modes of sight, hearing, and the somatic senses than we have of the so-called "chemical senses," or taste and smell. In any case, an aspect of

---

41 "Our senses represent the origin of the process of adaptation in continual dynamic equilibrium that allows us to survive and interact with the world" (Buiatti 2014, 13).
42 "One can survey a room from the outside, but the feeling of the space, the sense of the space must develop inside. The sensuousness of architecture is the physical sensation of space. Perceiving, scanning, apprehending space — all this is done with all our senses" (Bernhard Leitner in dialogue with Ulrich Conrads: 1985, 31).
43 "Atmosphere can be considered a unique spatial sense that integrates all five known senses in embodied movement" (Peri Bader 2015, 261).
44 For more detail, see the next section entitled "fifth property: atmosphere is kinaesthetic and haptic."

fundamental importance is to explain how the sensory qualities converge in a single perceptive act. This process, which is generally defined the *binding* problem, does not apply only to perception but also to the conjunction of the characteristics of the objects or spaces in the memories and other mental content. The question is extremely complicated, and not yet entirely resolved, despite there being different potential solutions formulated (Spence 2020).

Fourth property: atmosphere is multimodal

Besides multisensoriality, we speak of *sensorial multimodality*, a model that improves and exceeds that previously put forward as supramodality. The idea of multimodality rejects the existence of separate sensory modalities. Some scientists, having found the phenomenon in several areas of the brain, maintain that multimodal integration is "the norm" (Gallese and Lakoff 2005, 459). It happens that the firing of a single neuron can be correlated with different sensory modalities. "Sensory modalities like vision, touch, hearing, and so on are actually integrated with each other *and* with motor control and planning" (Gallese and Lakoff, 459: original italics).

Equally, it is possible to combine the hypothesis of *intermodality* to the perspective of multimodal functioning, in transcending the logic of strict modularity of sensory systems. It regulates the relationships between the signals produced contemporaneously in the different sensory modalities, allowing the association of a certain modality to sensations that it does not normally manage. This type of approach helps to explain how visual input (for example, textures and shapes) can contribute to the translation of tactile information (among which sensation of roughness and density). The phenomena of sensory intermodality can be reasonably interpreted as proof that information of a spatial nature has effects on different sensory modalities. For example, acoustic stimuli can influence the visual localisation of an object; more generally, the localisation of an object seems to be determined by a combination of sensory signs belonging to different modalities, with vision playing a preponderant role.

Fifth property: atmosphere is kinaesthetic and haptic

It's easy to say *touch*, relegating the expression to the action of touching with the hand. We read in the neuroscience textbooks that "the human hand is one of evolution's great creations" (Kandel et al. 2021, 435). The capacity to recognise an object exclusively on the basis of the touch of the hand is indeed one of the most important and complex functions of the somatosensory system. "When we are handed a baseball," for example, "we recognize it instantly without having to look at it because of its shape, size, weight, density, and texture" (Kandel et al., 436). The stimuli that are captured by the body's receptors do not only concern the extremities of the upper limbs but vast cutaneous areas, and are — in addition — very different to each other. There are five sensory modalities involved: touch (correlated to the perceptions of vibration, pressure, and cutaneous tension), proprioception,[45] pain, itching, and thermal sensitivity. The information gathered externally activates the cutaneous receptors in a highly selective and fragmentary manner; it is the central nervous system, where the sensory data are conveyed, along routes arranged in parallel, that manages the rejoining of the information coming from the periphery. The somatosensory cortex integrates and transforms this information into a unitary, coherent, and conscious tactile perception, gradually drawing out the identity-making characteristics of the stimulus.

The epidermis is the most extensive organ of the human body, but its tactile sensitivity is not homogenously distributed. There are areas of skin that are more active than others: on the basis of the density of peripheral innervation, it is possible to map a precise transposition of the peripheral receptor surface at a cerebral level, outlining the system of intracortical connections. This is the so-called *somatotopic map* (or *homunculus*), which should not be interpreted as a true portrayal of the body surface. The result is a distorted model of normal anatomical proportions, where the tips of the fingers, for example, are drawn in a cortical area quite a bit larger than that showing the back (Kandel et al. 2021, 84–85). This premise has been developed to highlight the capital role that information transmitted to the surface of the body — through all five solicited sensory modalities — plays in global spatial perception.

Although "buildings are appropriated in a twofold manner: by use and by perception — or rather, by touch and sight," as Walter Benjamin states ([1936] 2007, 240),[46] tactile fruition of spaces receives scant attention,

---

45 Proprioception (also known as kinaesthesia) is the faculty to perceive and recognise — without the support of sight — the position of one's own body in space, controlling its movements and the state of muscle contraction.
46 Very similar is the position of the architectural historian Kenneth Frampton: "the unavoidably earthbound nature of building is as tectonic and tactile in character

above all if one neglects the field of applied ergonomic design. To speak of tactile sensations in architecture implies two main assessments: 1. — entering the territory of criticism, advanced by some contemporary scholars (over whom Juhani Pallasmaa stands out), of the *oculocentric drift* that is infecting western architectural culture;[47] 2. — engaging with the theme of *hapticity*.[48] The first time I encountered this term, associated with atmospheric research, I thought it concerned an unknown concept while nonetheless having the sensation that I'd come across it somewhere before. At first I couldn't recall, but I was right: *haptic feedback* (also called *haptics*) is a function on iPhones, useful for providing information to the user in brief — almost imperceptible — vibrations. When managing the ringtone volume, I had come across the expression several times, although never dwelling too much on its meaning. In recent years a certain sensibility towards a haptic reading of physical space has gradually increased, promoted as much by philosophical as by architectural research. To introduce the idea of "haptic," I have chosen the definition Giuliana Bruno put forward in her *Atlas of Emotion*, at the start of the first decade of this millennium.

> As the Greek etymology tells us, haptic means "able to come into contact with." As a function of the skin, then, the haptic — the sense of touch — constitutes the reciprocal *contact* between us and the environment, both housing and extending communicative interface. But the haptic is also related to kinesthesis, the ability of our bodies to sense their own movement in space. (Bruno 2002, 6: original italics)

The sense of touch acquired its due autonomy and importance, in atmospheric logic, due to lending itself "in an existential sense," or as a sense of the experience localised in a precise place at a precise moment: "the actuality of existence, that is the essence of atmosphere" (Pallasmaa in response to Böhme: Böhme 2013d, 99). Equally, the anthropologist Tim Ingold (2012) finds a very close connection between the haptics and the atmospherics, maintaining that the operation of atmospheric stitching that every human being engenders with the structure of reality is intrinsically haptic. From the moment that "our contact with the world takes place

---

as it is scenographic and visual" (1995, 2).
47 See Eisenman 1992; Levin 1993; Pallasmaa 1994, 1998, 2012a, 2016b; Robinson 2012; Canepa 2017; Pérez Liebergesell, Vermeersch, and Heylighen 2019; Spence 2020.
48 See Pallasmaa 2000; O'Neill 2001; Mallgrave 2010; Papale et al. 2016.

at the boundary line of self through specialized parts of our enveloping membrane," for Juhani Pallasmaa "all the senses, including vision, are extensions of the tactile sense" (Pallasmaa and Zambelli 2020, 123). From this perspective, it is interesting to note the interpretation that the German art historian Wilhelm Worringer (1881–1965) gives to the concept of agoraphobia. Worringer highlights how the human being is naturally inclined to look for a contact of tactile perception with their physical environment, contact that completes the information on reality extractable through visual contemplation.

> In popular terms, [the] physical dread of open places may be explained as a residue from a normal phase of man's development, at which he was not yet able to trust entirely to visual impression as a means of becoming familiar with a space extended before him, but was still dependent upon the assurances of his sense of touch. As soon as man became a biped, and as such solely dependent upon his eyes, a slight feeling of insecurity was inevitably left behind. In the further course of his evolution, however, man freed himself from this primitive fear of extended space by habituation and intellectual reflection. *
> * In this context we may recall the fear of space which is clearly manifested in Egyptian architecture. The builders sought by means of innumerable columns, devoid of any constructional function, to destroy the impression of free space and to give the helpless gaze assurance of support by means of these columns. (Worringer [1908] 1997, 15–16 and n. 8)

The supposed supremacy of the sensory channel of touch in atmospheric perception is not currently acknowledged by scientific confirmation (Papale et al. 2016; Spence 2020). Effectively, beyond speculations of a critical-theoretical nature, however fascinating, "in humans, of all sensory modalities, vision is the most highly developed; over half of the cortex processes visual information" (Kandel et al. 2000, 427).

Sixth property: atmosphere is instinctive

Even with eyes closed, it is possible to feel the atmosphere in a room.

Some claim that "one mostly smells an atmosphere, breathes it in" (Griffero 2014a, 64), to the point of admitting the "atmospheric centrality of olfaction, or better of the 'oral sensorium' (olfaction and taste)" (Griffero, 66). As Tonino Griffero explains, the reasons are numerous: the senses of smell and taste are, firstly, involuntary and constant, indispensable for survival;[49] they are instinctive and violent in imposing their emotional charge, especially if activated by a trail welded to the memory, penetrated in the deepest unconscious and controllable with extreme difficulty.[50] The exploration of space through non-visual atmospheres is a visceral perceptual experience, which exemplifies the intuitive and immediate character of the atmospheric event. Actually, "in colloquial language one would probably answer the question as to how one perceives atmospheres as follows: 'by intuition. I just feel it'" (Böhme 1991, 35).

5. Atmospheric Bodies

"Architecture must not be static. It must possess, contain, and express a tension," writes Gio Ponti (1960, 187) in his wonderful book *In Praise of Architecture*. In the preceding chapters, I have shown how architecture, by means of the atmospheres it radiates, effuses a *perceptive tension*, which reflects on spatially immersed animate bodies. The choice of the word "bodies" is not random. "Atmosphere always and above all touches corporeality" (Griffero 2005a, 292). The requirement of *corporeality* alludes to two conditions: *having a body* and, at the same time, *being a body* (Wehrle 2020). In the resonance between architectural setting and perceiving subject is the body that first experiences the stimuli coming from what surrounds it, to then communicate — often without us being aware — how it is to find oneself in a certain atmosphere. This is a transition inside "the peculiar vagueness and the temporary disorientation that characterises the ingressive experience of atmospheres" (Böhme 2001, 88). That is, a sensation of instability and subsequent re-balancing, which grows in intensity if we come into contact with an artificial set that deliberately accentuates our emotional reactivity, as occurs when faced with a theatrical stage or exhibition room (Böhme 2013e).

According to Bruno Zevi, "the specific property of architecture — the feature distinguishing it from all other forms of art — consists in its working with a three-dimensional vocabulary which includes man" ([1948] 1993, 22). Architecture puts itself forward as "a great hollowed-out sculpture which man enters and apprehends by moving about within it" (Zevi, 22).

---

49   As much in respiration as in nutrition.
50   "We entrust ourselves entirely to our first experienced orosensory atmosphere, namely the maternal one, and we elevate it to territorial mark and later to condition of possibility for any subsequent atmosphere of trust" (Griffero 2014a, 68).

To exist as such, the architectural void necessitates the experience of a body, dynamically interactive and atmospherically receptive. Atmosphere cannot exist without the presence of a body that perceives it.[51] As Gernot Böhme clarifies, observing the work of figures like Peter Zumthor and Juhani Pallasmaa, "the introduction of the term 'atmosphere' leads to this redefinition of the art of architecture: architecture is the creation and design of spaces of corporeal presence" (2013d, 99). The question that spontaneously emerges is what do we mean by "body," when we talk about atmospheric processes.

The body is the founding nucleus that permits a total experience of architecture, capable of being embodied, integrated, multisensory, emotional, and prereflexive — hence: atmospheric. The basis is given by the anatomical presence, provided with sense organs and neural circuits, thanks to which the organism is able to gather and elaborate the stimuli produced by the external environment. Paradoxically, a potent manner of understanding the nature of our body is by imagining its absence. Indeed, "we are aware of having a body, in the pregnant, occlusive, onerous sense of corporeality, only when it or a part of it does not function properly" (Melandri 1968, 14). In a way, the *atmospheric body* is comparable to the infant body; a body that instinctively discovers its connection with the surrounding space and perceives atmospheric impressions by means of the senses and their synthesis, excited by the emotional traces that it receives. It is the body of an architect that doesn't know it is one yet, the body of a toddler Richard Neutra, learning the first — decisive — lessons on how to experience space.

> Early in life we spend much time floored baby-fashion, perplexed, most curious. As a two-and three-year-old, I often sat on the parquet of my parents' apartment, studying the raised, splintery grain of the worn hardwood and the warped boards. The cracks between the boards were filled with a compact something which I liked to dig out with my fingers. To grown-ups the floor is distant. Had they stooped to examine what I produced from this quiet resting place of open parquetry joints, they would have called it dirt. […] I tested it by the toddler's ancient test — put it into the mouth and found it 'no good.' Strange as it may seem, my first impressions of architecture were largely gustatory. […] I recall, that scantily dressed or naked as I was, I became uneasily aware of the surface on which I sat and moved. […] Our parlor ceiling was uncomfortably

---

51 One of the main (and few) points that those who study atmospheric dynamics, in various disciplinary fields, agree on is that an *unfelt atmosphere* does not exist (Osler and Szanto 2021).

high, and so I used to sit and play under the grand piano. The low headroom under our piano provided me the coziest place I knew. [...] Those many childhood experiences taught unspoken lessons in appreciation of space, texture, light, and shade, the smell of carpets, the warmth of wood, and the coolness of the stone hearth in front of our kitchen stove. (Neutra 1954, 25–26)

The *atmospheric body* is not just an anatomical presence, it is the root of experience. It is physical infrastructure, frontier of perception and awareness, but it is not any random somatic vector: it is the primordium of sensory contact of *a* particular subject, localised in *a* specific place, which permits their interaction with the outside world, allowing them to feel, act, and know. The biological matrix is completed by excerpts of personal experience that make an individual unique, and is influenced by the peculiar architectural characteristics that define the space in which we move.[52] In substance: a *Leib*, the felt body, lived body, that is the body sensed by the subject, the body that allows the subject to confer a meaning to received stimuli; the *Leib* that German phenomenologists distinguish — out of necessity of integration — from *Körper*, the biological body, which is the living material device. The neuroscientific approach (and that of the biological sciences, in a comprehensive sense) can make an important contribution to the interpretation of the relationship between the *lived body* (felt body) and the *living body* (material body), between *Leib* and *Körper*, between *being a body* and *having a body* (Shusterman 2006). It makes this double nature of our corporeality coexist, moving forward in the patrimony of acquired — and acquirable — notions on one of the two poles in particular: the *Körper*, of which the brain is a constituent part (Mallgrave and Gepshtein 2021).

> We are *Körper* (objectual and represented body) and *Leib* (lived body), as Edmund Husserl maintained. Today cognitive neuroscience can shed new light on the *Leib* by investigating the *Körper*. The point is not to reduce the *Leib* to the *Körper*, but to understand that the empirical investigation of the *Körper* can tell us new things about the *Leib*. (Gallese and Cuccio 2015, 19)

It is thanks to the *Körper* that we physically resonate with the atmosphere that diffuses in a place. Initially, there is "the atmospheric perception of an indeterminate presence," then atmosphere "abandons its originally synaesthetic nature" to show itself "in specific sensory performances,"

---

52 Principally, by the abovementioned *generators of atmosphere*. For more, see the section of the present chapter entitled "first property: atmosphere is composite."

potentially recognisable in distinct elements that can be mapped in space. It leads "symmetrically to the awareness of the subject of not being only felt body (*Leib*) but also material body (*Körper*), liable to be physically in agreement with it" (Griffero 2005a, 290).

Numerous external pressures act on our body, outpost to triggering atmospheric contact. Theories distilled from the modern biological sciences can open up singular (and perhaps unexpected) horizons on the mutual dependence that exists between architectonically organised spaces and the instinctive reactions of people immersed in those spaces.[53] Namely: it is important to understand if and how evolutionary plasticity[54] and cognitive pressures, induced by the cultural parabola and technological shock, can share in the mechanisms of perception of the architectural substance. The discussion of the atmospheric phenomenon hinges on this axis of mediation, strenuously balanced between impulses released by genetic legacy and demiurgic influence deployed by the external context, understood as much as a physical environment as a socio-cultural and familiar milieu, in which the organism grows and is formed.

In summarising the full circuit of existing relations, we come to the conclusion that "we are embodied beings whose minds, bodies, environment, and culture are interconnected at sundry levels" (2013, 7). Harry Francis Mallgrave, author of the above assertion, which might appear obvious to many readers, also states that "its far-reaching implications have only begun to be fully appreciated in the last few years — prompted, as it were, by the many dramatic discoveries and breakthroughs of the biological sciences" (2013, 7). The key idea is that there is a solid and dynamic integration of parts, in which "the brain, the body, and the environment are in effect codetermining of each other and therefore coevolving" (Mallgrave 2015a, 30). The atmospheric tension emphasizes this close interconnection, outlining *a continuum of emotions, body, brain, mind, space, and architecture*,[55] which proves to be inherently tied to the individual physiology of the aesthetic-perceptive experience. We could define this reading of the human being as "biological embodiment," a sort of evolutionary mutation of the phenomenological legacy, celebratory

---

53 It is fundamental to remember that "all behaviors are shaped by the interplay of genes and the environment" (Kandel et al. 2021, 26).
54 "Genes that are stably inherited over generations create the machinery by which new experiences can change the brain during learning" (Kandel et al. 2021, 26).
55 Architecture as a cultural product of human activity.

of the primacy of the human experience, on which operate insights for reflection provided by the biological sciences (Petitot et al. 1999).

The concept of *embodiment* has attracted great enthusiasm over the last thirty or so years,[56] during which "scholars followed divergent paths in search of a definition none of which touched upon embodied understanding" unanimously (Iran-Nejad and Irannejad 2017, 2). The initial intent was to replicate the paradigms of a reductionist, dualist, computational, and representational stamp of the very first season of classical cognitive science.[57] The fundamental premise consists in recognising that individual and environment are so closely interconnected and interdependent with each other that it is impossible to think of them as autonomous dualistically opposed realities. Perception and cognition have their origin from the living organism, to be considered a single entity that includes the environment in which it lives within the confines of its existence. In modern literature, a large number of models and explanations have been deployed to analyse the unit of identity between the perceiving subject and their context of interaction; recently, an expression has been coined to gather together and order this composite vein of research: *4EA cognitive science*, paradigm for which "cognition is enactive, embodied, embedded, affective and (potentially) extended" (Ward and Stapleton 2012, 89). At times it is held that these approaches are broadly complementary, at others that they produce theories that are basically incompatible. The intense emphasis on the body-environment unit and the strong continuity of thought with phenomenological teaching[58] is stimulating even within the architectural

---

56 The beginning of the history of *embodied cognition* dates back to the publication of the volume *The Embodied Mind* (Varela, Thompson, and Rosch 1991).
57 Cognitive science came into being back in the fifties, although the disciplines that make it up are much older and the heart of their research, *cognition*, already inspired philosophical debate in the time of the great Greek thinkers. Since "the comprehensive understanding of the human mind requires an organismic perspective" (Damasio 1994, 252), cognitive science possesses an inherently interdisciplinary structure, founded — by convention — on six constituent contributions: artificial intelligence, psychology, philosophy, linguistics, anthropology, and neuroscience (Gardner 1985; Bermúdez 2020).
58 We arrive at the positions synthesised above by passing through the domain of so-called *neurophenomenology*, a methodological remedy for the "hard problem" of human experience, put forward by the Chilean philosopher and neuroscientist Francisco Javier Varela García (1946–2001), at the end of the last century. "Neurophenomenology is the name I am using [...] to designate a quest to marry modern cognitive science and a *disciplined approach* to human experience, thus placing

discipline[59] the adoption of models informed by the enactive-embodied cognition perspective (Jelić and Staničić 2020), as "a basis of neuroscientific and phenomenological interpretation of architectural experience" (Jelić et al. 2016, 1). The objective is to return human experience to the centre of architectural design and research: attention is on the "pre-reflective" dimension of the architectural process (Jelić 2015), in which to explore the embodied nature of atmospheric contact, as the precognitive two-way interaction between an architectonic work and the body.[60]

6. The Swarm of Emotions

The third contribution, after multisensorial dynamics and embodied experience, which proves fundamental at the triggering of the atmospheric impulse, is made up of emotional echoes guiding spatial perception. Architecture, is, in effect "a phenomenon of the emotions, lying outside questions of construction and beyond them," asserts Le Corbusier. Then he clarifies that "the purpose of construction is TO MAKE THINGS HOLD TOGETHER; of architecture TO MOVE US" (1931, 19: original small capitals). Every aspect of architectonic matter, detectable "in the very bones of the buildings, not in the trimmings only," if it is a manifestation of the "human factor" (Gropius [1937] 1962, 88), exerts influences of an emotional nature, "both on the level of our coupling with the built environment […] and in how our design mediates or fosters our socio-cultural interactions with others" (Mallgrave 2015a, 31).

The emotional value of the architectural experience is expressed through the atmospheres it produces. The atmospheres are entrusted with the job of evoking and amplifying the emotions ignited in the individual by the sensory findings of the spatial medium in which they are immersed. The first contact that is established with the architectural surroundings is of emotional origin: so it is immediate and preconscious, managed by physiological and neural mechanisms, that precede any discussion about

---

      myself in the lineage of the continental tradition of phenomenology" (Varela 1996, 330: original italics).
59 Over the centuries, inspired at first by Vitruvian theses, the architectural theory evolved several notions of *embodiment* (Pasqualini, Llobera, and Blanke 2013).
60 This approach also challenges the dominance of bodily reductive conceptions in architecture (Imrie 2003).

rational control; which is to say, an atmospheric impression comes to life by pure *emotional instinct*.

We perceive atmosphere through our emotional sensibility — a form of perception that works incredibly quickly, and which we humans evidently need to help us survive. Not every situation grants us time to make up our minds on whether or not we like something or whether indeed we might be better heading off in the opposite direction. (Zumthor 2006, 13)

Such automatism of interaction with the physical environment has biological bases and is, in great part, determined by one's own evolutionary structure, besides attitudes assimilated from the social milieu or the family context in which one has grown up. It seems, states Juhani Pallasmaa, that "we are genetically and culturally conditioned to seek or avoid certain types of situations or atmospheres" (2014a, 233). Generally, in the past, there has been a tendency to underestimate the perceptual role of the emotions in codifying the characteristics of a designed space, often considering them "trivial," in favour of rational knowledge, held up by arguments of a conceptual or verbal order. "But actually their effect upon men's actions is immense," asserts Sigfried Giedion (1954, 426), among the most important architecture historians and critics of the twentieth century (1888–1968).[61] "The scope and strength of the emotions are both greater than we sometimes suppose" (Giedion, 426): first of all, emotions are capable of — instantaneously — providing more comprehensive and synthetic evaluations on the whole collection of stimuli acting on the sentient subject with respect to any other form of analysis. From an evolutionary point of view, emotions represent physiological responses that arise, independently of the reason's supervision, to optimise the vital processes and the actions that every organism undertakes in their environment — hence, with architecture itself.

At this point, a clarification is essential: the term "emotion" should be understood, in this context of research, in its biological sense. The emotions, besides being conceptualised ideals, possess a physically based and scientifically explicable correlate. A condition that is certainly not overlooked by designers, who are well aware of how "the emotions that architecture arouses spring from physical conditions which are

---

61 After graduating in engineering, Giedion studies history of art in Munich, where he earns his doctorate under the auspices of Heinrich Wölfflin (cf. Frampton 1995, n. 3). See the section of this chapter entitled "empathy and architecture."

inevitable [and] irrefutable" (Le Corbusier 1931, 26). Emotions should be considered for what they are congenitally: "cellular signals that are involved in the process of translating information into physical reality, [...] at the nexus between matter and mind, going back and forth between the two and influencing both" (Pert 1997, 189). Such signals douse the living organism: they are produced by the nervous system, in that they are "an interplay between higher brain centers and subcortical regions such as the hypothalamus and amygdala" that translates into "the emotional experiences that we perceive as fear, anger, pleasure, and contentment" (Kandel et al. 2000, 996).

There are three contributions that, although they can be studied independently, mutually influence each other in the assembly of emotions: 1. — a repertoire of *compensatory changes*, coordinated by three physiological systems (the endocrine glands, the autonomic nervous system, and the musculoskeletal system);[62] 2. — behavioural action that is manifested in *motor and expressive outputs* (both facial and bodily); 3. — the conscious experience of the felt emotional state (that takes the name of *feeling*). This explanation accounts for emotions as a complex combination of regulatory and cognitive functions, defined by relative changes in physiology, behaviour, and feelings, which help human beings to respond in a flexible manner to *biologically significant environmental stimuli*. It thus implies admitting that emotions determine physiological and behavioural effects that, even when they are not consciously accessible, are subjectable to scientific enquiry (Delplanque and Sander 2021).

Once the neurobiological foundation of emotional phenomena is grasped, we should clarify the lexicon adopted when we speak of emotions: it is common to use words having precise meanings as though they were synonyms.[63] The first observation concerns the terms *emotion* and *feeling*.

---

62 "The endocrine system is responsible for the secretion and regulation of hormones into the bloodstream that affect bodily tissues and the brain. The autonomic system mediates changes in the various physiological control systems of the body: the cardiovascular system, the visceral organs, and the tissues in the body cavity. The skeletal motor system mediates overt behaviors such as freezing, fight-or-flight, and particular facial expressions. Together, these three systems control the physiological expression of emotion states in the body" (Kandel et al. 2021, 1045–1046).

63 "Theories of emotion are as old as psychology itself, or even older, and many different attempts at conceptualizing and measuring emotions have been made" (Küller et al. 2006, 1504). Although emotional dynamics have long been studied,

An emotional state has two components, one evident in a characteristic physical sensation and the other as a conscious feeling — we sense our heart pounding *and* we consciously feel afraid. To maintain the distinction between these two components, the term "emotion" sometimes is used to refer only to the bodily state (i.e., the emotional state) and the term "feeling" is used to refer to conscious sensation. (Kandel et al. 2000, 983: original italics)

The exterior manifestation of emotion is defined *affect* and can be made clear in different ways: through changes to facial expression, posture, and gesture, through inflexions of the vocal tone, or through autonomic symptoms[64] (such as emotional lacrimation and an increase in salivation). To guarantee the adequate adaptive plasticity, requested by an environment in continual transformation, emotional states have quite a compressed duration: emotions are immediate, developing in milliseconds — a speed too fast to be consciously perceived and interpreted; feelings come a bit later, ignited by cognition. If the parabola of an emotional state continues in time, going beyond the threshold of extemporaneity, it constitutes a *mood*. Lastly, we can speak of *character*, or rather the range of ordinary tendencies — induced by both experiential and genetic factors — that drive an individual to react to emotional situations in a positive or negative way, shaping the construction of their personality.

In recent years, we have seen notable progress in the understanding of the neurophysiological correlates of emotions, an extremely complex field of research, which must be confronted as much with ethical questions[65] as methodological limitations[66]. In addition, the issue emerges of the subjective nature of the emotional experience, whose analysis is generally entrusted to self-assessment formulas, of limited reliability. Measures of this type are sensitive to individual factors hard to control (such as the instability

---

there are no univocal definitions. A review written in the early eighties identifies more than ninety meanings in emotion literature (Kleinginna and Kleinginna 1981).

64   Relative, that is, to the *autonomic nervous system*. This coordinates somatic, emotional, and behavioural responses of the organism in order to regulate its *homeostasis*, which maintains at optimal levels the essential physiological processes (such as heartbeat, blood pressure, and respiratory rate). Due to its functional characteristics, the autonomic nervous system is able to give prompt integrated responses to variations in the external environment.

65   Tied to the risk of compromising the emotional balance of subjects undergoing experiments that anticipate interference in their affective sphere.

66   Technologies currently available, both neurophysiological testing and neurofunctional imaging, do not yet allow for the necessary accuracy in recording emotional activity mediated by deep subcortical structures.

and emotional fluctuation of examined subjects) and to social factors (such as the presence of the examiner). Despite these obstacles, interest in scientific research into emotions is advancing appreciably, including in the observation of the emotional impact of architectural design (Bower, Tucker, and Enticott 2019).

Neuropsychological studies have identified the existence of hemispheric asymmetries in the governance of emotion, suggesting for example the so-called *right-hemisphere hypothesis*, which asserts (on the basis of scientific evidence) that "the right hemisphere is more intimately concerned with both the perception and expression of emotions than is the left hemisphere" (Purves et al. 2018, 717); it oversees the assimilation of visual and auditory input with emotional relevance, as indeed the emotional production of facial mimicry and the prosody of speech.[67] Sustained by experimental findings in which it is noticed that "the right hemisphere is specialized for (among other things) visuospatial and emotional processing" (Purves et al., 752), Juhani Pallasmaa considers that "the recognition of atmospheric entities takes place in a peripheral and subconscious manner primarily through the right hemisphere"[68] (2014a, 238). This is, obviously, a speculative supposition, synthesized by a theorist from the architectural discipline, lacking (for the moment) any scientific endorsement, which assumes value mainly for its aim to articulate new queries, providing original insights for reflection and experimentation on atmospheric dynamics.

For a long time, research into emotions of a neurobiological stamp has been profitably accompanied by psychological knowledge, which has helped to better clarify the neural roots of emotional behaviour. Among the most important explanatory models that have been perfected, we recall *categorical theories* and *dimensional theories*. The first, in interpreting the emotions as discreet entities, distinguishing two emotional classes: *basic emotions*, which are innate, "pan-cultural, evolutionarily old, shared with other species, and expressed by a particular physiological pattern and facial configuration;" and *complex emotions*, which are learnt over the course of development, "socially and culturally shaped, evolutionarily new, and typically expressed by a combination of the response patterns

---

67 By the term "prosody" we mean the collection of tonal modulations, rhythmic patterns, and accents that accompany sounds emitted during speech. In substance, it supplies emotional information for speech.
68 The reference, in particular, is the thesis about the "divided brain" formulated by the British psychiatrist Iain McGilchrist ([2009] 2019).

that characterize basic emotions" (Purves et al. 2012, glossary). The selection of the basic emotions[69] has not been precisely codified, either in numerical terms or in nature, due to the extreme difficulty of probing the immense repertoire of human emotional reactions, in all their expressive and functional nuances. The operation is further complicated, as is easy to predict, in the study of complex emotions (for example, pride and nostalgia), since these derive from the composition of primary emotions and are contaminated by a greater rate of interference as a result of intercultural differences.

An alternative approach to categorical theories is made up of the dimensional perspective: this profiles the emotions as points along a continual flow, oscillating between two or more critical dimensions in the emotional space. There are many, arbitrarily legitimable, parameters that can be chosen to describe emotions, but two components are considered fundamental by the most part of researchers; namely: *arousal*, which defines the physiological and/or subjective intensity of the emotion; and *valence*, which evaluates the direction of the emotion in terms of hedonic quality.[70] This last model of detection and representation of the emotional states has already been tested to analyse the emotional genesis of the atmospheric perception within preliminary experimental experiences (Canepa et al. 2018, 2019).

Cyclically, hypotheses have been put forward regarding the existence of emotional propensions innate to the human genetic constitution, due to the instinct for self-preservation. Harry Francis Mallgrave, in his book *Architecture and Embodiment*, cites the case of the psychological theories of Professor Richard Coss (2003), who examined "several evolutionary templates of visual behavior (fixed-action patterns) and their biological responses (visual releasers), among them [...] our emotional preference for rounded versus pointed patterns" (2013, 153). According to his thesis, to know "such visual preferences [...] probably born of predation (eluding threats to our survival), as well as of social signalling with a view toward sexual selection" (Mallgrave, 153), that is to understand the code of biological programming in human beings, would help to direct the emotional reactions researched by architects and artists.

---

69 Conventionally identified in anger, fear, sadness, disgust, happiness, and surprise.
70 Emotions, apart from more differentiation, are intrinsically pleasant or unpleasant (Barrett et al. 2007).

In reality, "architecture should not specify emotion, but should invite emotion" (Havik and Tielens 2013b, 43). This observation recalls the etymology of the term "emotion," which, as Giuliana Bruno highlights, has a very close relationship with the idea of movement.

> The Latin root of the word "emotion" speaks clearly about a "moving" force, stemming as it does from *emovere*, an active verb composed of *movere*, "to move," and *e*, "out." The meaning of emotion, then, is historically associated with "a moving out, migration, transference from one place to another." (Bruno 2002, 6: original italics)

The emotional potential injected into the body of architecture should imply instinctive feedback, likely to titillate the atmospheric sensitivity, without necessarily leading — as sometimes occurs — to a stereotypical accentuation of the built environment's atmosphere or to its interpretation in a pre-eminently aesthetic-visual category. In the first case, intending to amplify the outbreak of emotions, some architects arrive at the design of smart atmospheric machines, sophisticatedly elaborated to shape emotional landscapes, synthetic and enriched, in which all the user's senses are involved in an interplay of electrical, light, smell, and sound components. Many examples can be seen in contemporary parametric and biomorphic architecture. such as the experimental exhibition set-up, *Hylozoic Ground*, ideated by Philip Beesley for the Canada Pavilion at the 12th International Architecture Exhibition in Venice (Ohrstedt and Isaacs 2010). At the same time, there is the possibility we may run a further risk: compressing and flattening the emotional charge of the atmospheric resource at a level solely of the visual system, deputing it as preponderant aesthetic catalyser of the emotional potential. Alberto Pérez-Gómez brings out this problem well, underlining how "interest in atmosphere in the visual arts and architecture [...] is associated with aesthetic effects in presentation drawings, buildings, and installations" (2016, 16). He looks into the possible reasons.

> Perhaps surprisingly, the impoverishment of the qualitative and emotive living environment in cities was an important motivation behind the late-eighteenth-century recognition of character and atmospheres as visual aesthetic categories. (Pérez-Gómez 2016, 15)

Atmospheric qualities, detonators of emotional stimuli, as much poetical as physiological, can be traced back to those architectural solutions that, shaking up a complex and active assemblage of forces, prove to be capable — also in a manner that is not fully aware — of encouraging the development of an attunement, variously intoned and not rigidly pre-packaged. There is no necessity to turn to artificially intricate tectonics. It is the unity of details, bearers of atmospheric effects, that arouses the *swarm of emotions* that capture the individual. A master of atmosphere like Peter Zumthor is well aware of this: "the perfectly tempered feel of his built spaces is immediately communicated to viewers, residents, visitors and the immediate neighbourhood" (Labs-Ehlert 2005, 7). This is how Zumthor reflects on the emotional power of atmospheric environments:

> So what moved me? Everything. The things themselves, the people, the air, noises, sound, colours, material presences, textures, forms too — forms I can appreciate. Forms I can try to decipher. Forms I find beautiful. What else moved me? My mood, my feelings, the sense of expectation that filled me while I was sitting here. Which brings that famous Platonic sentence to mind: "beauty is in the eye of the beholder." Meaning: it is all in me. But then I perform an experiment. I take away the square — and my feelings are not the same. An elementary experiment, certainly — please excuse the simplicity of my thinking. I remove the square and my feelings disappear. I could never have had those feelings without the atmosphere of the square. It's quite logical really. People interact with objects. (Zumthor 2006, 17)

7. Empathic Contagion

The definition of atmosphere as a condition of emotional resonance and potential consonance between the perceiving subject and their architectonic surroundings has a very important corollary, as stated at the beginning of the chapter. In other words, it is supposed that within this *atmospheric continuum* an empathic connection develops between the animate subject (the sentient individual) and the inanimate object (the surrounding architectonic space). Before going on to explain the empathic appendix of the perceptual atmospheric event, it is worth mentioning some preliminary (though minor) notions.

Empathy and architecture

To speak of *empathy* implies going into an issue as complex, versatile, and elusive as that of atmosphere. Perhaps even more so, since it has been studied systematically and in depth for a good deal longer,[71] tackled — in

---

[71] Resurfaced in the contemporary debate about human cognition after decades of "almost complete oblivion" (Gallese 2003a, 172).

parallel — by numerous disciplines, scientific, humanistic, and artistic. It is hard to identify with clarity a single semantic direction (Lanzoni 2018). Initially, the concept of *Einfühlung* came into being, generally translated as "empathy,"[72] although its original meaning (literally "feeling into") alludes to the act of projecting oneself onto another body, not necessarily human, like a work of art or a spatial configuration. The term *Einfühlung* was coined in the second half of the nineteenth century by Robert Vischer ([1873] 1994), German historian and philosopher of art, recognised by Benedetto Croce ([1934] 1967) as the father of the theory of empathy, and acquired renown thanks to the publication of *Abstraction and Empathy* ([1908] 1997),[73] the seminal work by Wilhelm Worringer.[74]

Empathy is a later English translation of the word *Einfühlung*, put forward by the British psychologist Edward Titchener (1909), a pupil of Wilhelm Wundt, the figure considered the founder of modern experimental psychology. The Greek etymon is located in the annexing of the preposition ἐν (*en*), or "in," to the noun πάθεια (*pátheia*), derived from the theme παθ- of the verb πάσχω (*pásko*), which means "to suffer" or "to endure." Today, the word *empathy* is widely used in common language, and is often a source of incomprehension and semantic variation due to its malleable interpretability. The parabola of the empathic theorem has alternated, from its formulation, between phases of intense interest and cycles of stasis: "ensnared by the accusation of being an irrationalistic theme and overly indebted to nineteenth century biology and psychology," this "is brusquely interrupted by the advent of a new philosophical current, phenomenology, which in the first decade of the twentieth century revolutionises the study of consciousness" (Boella 2006, 3). Despite the gradual loss of interest among art historians and in the field of psychology, enquiry into the empathic dynamics "lingered for decades within the discourse of modern architecture" (Koss 2006, 139).

For some years now, the investigation into the feeling of empathy has returned to the centre of academic attention, regaining the impetus of the original corporeal-physiological perspective (Pasqualini and Blanke 2014),

---

72 Being a word of extremely wide-ranging and complex meaning (see Spitzer 1942a, 1942b, 1963), there are many similar expressions such as "sympathy," "compassion," or "understanding," which over time have commingled and substituted each other.
73 Original title: *Abstraktion und Einfühlung*.
74 For a historic overview of the concept, see Nowak 2011; Curtis and Elliott 2014.

which proved to be particularly compatible with recent neuroscientific discoveries and theories of the mind. As Francisco Varela observes, one of the key figures in the current season of the (neuro)phenomenological reintegration of empathy, the ferment could usefully be explained through "various parallel empirical studies, that is, some of its natural correlates from scientific studies rather than [phenomenological reduction] itself" (1996, 340 n. 7). This has led to a return to the reflections of authors such as Adolf von Hildebrand (1847–1921), Theodor Lipps (1851–1914), August Schmarsow (1853–1936), Heinrich Wölfflin (1864–1945), Aby Warburg (1866–1929), and August Endell (1871–1925). Given the themes addressed, directly concerning the area of architectural discipline, noteworthy — for their improbable relevance today[75] — are the analytical intuitions of the Swiss art historian Heinrich Wölfflin, which provide the roots to a potential *primitive theory of empathy in the architectural experience*.

> *Our own bodily organization is the form through which we apprehend everything physical.* I shall now show that the basic elements of architecture — material and form, gravity and force — are defined by our experiences of ourselves; that the laws of formal aesthetics are none other than the sole conditions under which our organic well-being appears possible; and, finally, that the expression intrinsic to horizontal and vertical articulation is presented according to human (organic) principles. (Wölfflin [1886] 1994, 157–158: original italics)

For scholars active in the field of architecture, *empathy* is, first and foremost, *the building up of a connection*, in which the architectonic work constitutes the element of mediation between the architect's imagination and the occupant's experience.[76] The architect must show proof of possessing, even without fully controlled rationality, as if moved by an innate instinct, the ability to anticipate and invent the future of spaces to be prefigured (Buchert 2021). In particular, architects must be able to outline and tune — when the creative process is only at an embryonic state — the *general*

---

75 However inevitably immature and naive, tied to an approach "a little primitive, theoretically feeble, unfortunately still projectivistic and at times even grotesque in its associations (weight—nostalgia, symmetry—wellbeing, windows—eyes, round arch—happiness, etc.)" (Griffero 2014a, 94).

76 "As you are designing, you are always shifting back and forth between evaluating and imaging. [...] We 'orchestrate' the imagined experience. [...] Orchestrating the experience entails making every design choice come together into a whole — an interaction gestalt. [...] We have to *live* our designs, repeatedly, during the design process" (Höök 2018, 99–100: original italics).

atmosphere that will qualify built environments; this operation is "the most ephemeral and complex of [all] subconscious mental simulations" that they must accomplish, "because an atmosphere or ambiance is not an object, but something suspended between the setting and the subject" (Pallasmaa 2014b, 76). One could even maintain that the essential component of any architectural act conscious of its meaning originates from the architect's empathic imagination, being the organ of calibration and orchestration of all the future emotional, cognitive, and motor contributions. To design a building, the architect must turn into the individual who will inhabit their spaces, as though designing for themselves: "a true architect does not design for a client at all as an external 'other,'" clarifies Juhani Pallasmaa. "He/she internalizes his/her client, as well as all the physical and logistic parameters, and designs for him/herself in his/her internalized role as the client" (Pallasmaa and Zambelli 2020, 101).

The introspective and simulative process, which is initiated between the empathic sensibility of the designer and that of the user, can even be explored the other way around. The end-user tends to reconnoitre the environment to seek out and unearth the intentions of whoever set up the scene with which they interact.

> We unconsciously look at things as if they had been produced by a human maker; [...] viewing hand-formed pottery, or the lines of a draftsman, or the lettering of a calligraphist, we unconsciously identify ourselves with their makers: we seem to follow vicariously the imagined muscular exertion in the nervous experience of the craftsman, as if experiencing it ourselves. (Neutra 1954, 74)

Yet again, the words of Richard Neutra appear extraordinarily groundbreaking, capable of foreshadowing the most current empathic theses elaborated on a physiological basis, to the extent that they seem to paraphrase the content of the so-called *embodied simulation* model.[77] As Harry Francis Mallgrave highlights, "the fact that occupants of a building also read the presumed intentions of architects, whether they are intentional or not, is in itself not a novel insight" (2013, 162).

> In their work architects generally expect their intentions to be read by the occupants of their buildings. But the fact that so much of this reading may take place at a precognitive level — different from reflectively attributing to

---

77 See the last section in the present chapter entitled "embodied simulation."

others the symbolic representation of intentions, beliefs, or attitudes — defines a crucial distinction that separates embodied simulation from earlier attempts to imbue a design with meaning. (Mallgrave 2013, 162)

In conclusion, the empathic imagination of the architect is a form of comprehension of the architectural experience in its entirety and multifocality, or rather, in its atmospheric nature. The atmosphere, which a place emanates and thanks to which the place establishes a perceptual relationship with those who live it, becomes a *medium of empathic contagion*, permeated with the magma of sensory stimuli, which, diffused from the architectonic body, spray the receptive interface of our organism. The threshold between internal and external dissolves, just as the confines between the dominion of subjective sensitivity and that of objective substance, between the animate body and inanimate material, lose stability.

Around the end of the nineteenth century, the hypothesis of empathic connection with inanimate space acquired explicit autonomy (Mallgrave and Ikonomou 1994; Mallgrave 2013). Robert Vischer, who, as explained above, brought to light the neologism *Einfühlung* ([1873] 1994), was the first author to extend the empathic reflection to theoretical questions of an architectural stamp. The evaluations that preliminarily emerged focused on the study of plastic forms; "applied to architecture, empathy was to be fruitful in enriching the concept of 'form' in the 1890s," states Adrian Forty (2000, 159). Heinrich Wölfflin, one of the theorists who had majorly inspired the diffusion and use of the empathic resource in architecture, offered an anthropomorphic concept of built space, in which our empathic response with the context is justified in terms of *somatic analogies*; a response, induced by architectural forms, fuelled by emotional instincts.

Some might become dubious and question what similarities or expressive feelings we could possibly share with an inanimate stone. Briefly, there are degrees of heaviness, balance, hardness, etc., all of which have expressive value for us. Since only the human form, of course, can express all that lies in humanity, architecture will be unable to express particular emotions that are manifested through specific faculties. Nor should it try to do so. Its subject remains the *great vital feelings*, the moods that presuppose a constant and stable body condition. Powerful columns energetically stimulate us; our respiration harmonizes with the expansive or narrow nature of the space. In the former case we are stimulated as if we ourselves were the supporting columns; in the latter case we breathe as deeply and fully as if our chest were as wide as the hall. Asymmetry is often experienced as physical pain, as if a limb were missing or injured. Likewise, we know the disagreeable condition that is induced by looking at something unbalanced, and so on. (Wölfflin [1886] 1994, 152; 154–155: original italics)

A few years later, in 1893, the German art historian August Schmarsow (1994), Heinrich Wölfflin's academic counterpart, formulated his version of the empathic phenomenon in the plastic dimension, in which he recognised the primacy of the spatial experience on form, analysing the close interdependence that he assumed exists between space and body. Space can be considered an imaginary but necessary extension of the body, without which it could not be perceived. The spatial experience is concretised in a nonconscious act of embodied dilation and projection, which generates a compound of corporeal modulations in response to the formal and material characteristics of the elements that populate the architectonic scene. In other words, the body, with its marked expressivity (managed through posture, facial mimicry, and motor responsiveness, as well as by means of autonomic nervous reactions), acts as a vehicle to mediate the expressivity that the subject reads in the architectonic aggregate. The body changes according to the environment in which it finds itself, and that happens without the possibility of exerting any control over it.

> The intuited form of space, which surrounds us wherever we may be and which we then always erect around ourselves and consider more necessary than the form of our own body, consists of the residues of sensory experience to which the muscular sensations of our body, the sensitivity of our skin, and the structure of our body all contribute. As soon as we have learned to experience ourselves and ourselves alone as the center of this space, whose coordinates intersect in us, we have found the precious kernel [...] on which architectural creation is based. (Schmarsow [1893] 1994, 286–287)

With August Schmarsow's theoretical position, decidedly less affected by forced formalism with respect to Heinrich Wölfflin's aesthetics, the empathic phenomenon assumes a more psychological intonation, anchored to a lesser degree to physiological aspects. A further evolution of the empathic dynamics towards the frontiers of psychological doctrine can be found in Theodor Lipps (1897, 1906), "who became the principal theorist of empathy theory at the turn of the century" (Mallgrave 2013, 125), so much so that he had a highly important influence on the formation of architects, although he himself never studied pre-eminently the architectural topic. Space, veritable catalyser of aesthetic perception, despite being that only if "ignited" by the sensitivity of the perceiving subject, becomes interacting substance that can be, not only observed, but also felt and shared. Human beings prove to have an innate propensity to animate unconsciously entire buildings and single architectural elements, projecting their own feelings onto them. A process of emotional co-participation and mimetic self-identification is triggered — understood as visceral psychological states, mobilised by a deep consonance between subject and object. The shift with respect to the intrinsically corporeal perspective, inaugurated by Robert Vischer, is strengthened. It will be the theoretical work of August Endell ([1908] 2018; 1995) to translate the spatial paradigm of empathic dynamics into more comprehensible and efficient terms for architects.

> Spatial structures in bodily experience, architectural forms as movements, architecture as the design of emptiness — with these concepts, Wölfflin, Schmarsow and Endell inaugurated a potential that has in no way been exhausted yet. (Böhme 2017b, 83–84)

Visuomotor resonance mechanisms

The development of the empathic theory proceeds over the years, promoting different positions: approaches switch between, for example, the formal, intellectualised, technological, and semiotic. However, this is not the place to take on such a digression,[78] which would end up taking a collateral tangent. What is of interest is to understand *what empathy means for architectural research in the contemporary era*, in the light of the notable level of experimental advance reached by the sciences of the mind (Leiberg and Anders 2006). Harry Francis Mallgrave points out "what was missing from theories of Einfühlung at the start of the twentieth century was a scientific basis to explain or to demonstrate in a definitive way how it is that we [...] empathize with the forms of our built environment" (2013, 133). To date, progress in understanding our biological and embodied roots gives us encouraging assumptions. It is interesting to note the circular trajectory of the evolution of theories on empathy: the starting point, marked by the early premises of a corporeal-physiological type, is joined by the current hypotheses developed in the research scenario opened up to the discovery of mirror neurons, which it is thought can offer neurological proof of our empathic relationship with the world (Newman 2018).

For several years now, the locution *mirror neurons* bounced in and out of the (neuro)scientific debate, eliciting great interest as much among

---

78 Only considering scientific literature written in English, we find more than forty definitions of "empathy" (Cuff et al. 2016).

experts as non-specialist public, to the extent that there are numerous warnings to avoid exaggerations in their divulgation (Hickok 2014); the attraction of this theme has aroused enthusiasm for nearly three decades,[79] when in the early nineties their existence was inadvertently discovered in a cycle of experiments performed at the Institute of Human Physiology of the University of Parma, directed by Professor Giacomo Rizzolatti.[80] It was a case of good fortune, because Rizzolatti's team,[81] while working on the premotor cortex of a group of macaques (a species, like men, with an eminently socio-relational nature), noticed the presence of a particular type of neuron, in the rostral part of the inferior premotor cortex (area F5): these neurons were found to activate selectively not only when the animal carried out a given action, for a certain purpose, such as grabbing food with their hand or breaking it in their mouth (a well-known fact), but also — in an entirely "unexpected" manner (Di Pellegrino et al. 1992, 179) — when the primate passively observed identical or analogous actions performed by the experimenters. Due to the specular nature of their response, this class of neurons was named *mirror neurons*.[82]

The next step was to ascertain their existence in man as well — a context of investigation that is undoubtedly more complex. A series of studies carried out in vivo using different experimental methods, among which behavioural, neurophysiological, and brain imaging techniques (Buccino, Binkofski, and Riggio 2004), demonstrated that an equivalent mechanism of *visuomotor resonance* is also present in the human brain: it was found

---

[79] The enthusiasm for this discovery and its potential gradually increased in the first decade of the 2000s, while today we are seeing an inflexion due to the difficulty of finding the necessary confirmations to validate the knowledge acquired with the first experiments. A rapid observation of the parabola of studies conducted on mirror neurons can be carried out by examining the stream of indexed publications in the archive of biomedical scientific literature *PubMed* (www.pubmed.ncbi.nlm.nih.gov). Inserting "mirror neuron" in the research search string and including both abstract and full paper, it appears that, after remaining on the threshold of twenty articles per annum during the nineties, the peak was reached in 2013 with more than two hundred and fifty contributions, to record less than half that in 2020. Similar results emerge when interrogating other sources, such as the database *Scopus* (Heyes and Catmur 2021).
[80] The first report on the discovery of mirror neurons was published in 1992 (Di Pellegrino et al. 1992).
[81] Made up of, among others, Vittorio Gallese, Luciano Fadiga, and Leonardo Fogassi.
[82] For a panoramic overview of the topic, see Ferrari and Rizzolatti 2014; Rizzolatti and Fogassi 2014.

to have populations of mirror neurons localised in various cortical regions (among which the premotor cortex and Broca's area). "So, when we observe a hand grasping an apple, the same population of neurons that control the execution of grasping movements becomes active in the observer's motor areas" (Rizzolatti, Fogassi, and Gallese 2001, 661). This means that we do not just see through our visual system (as was traditionally thought), but we also use our motor system; which is to say: the visual experience that we have of reality implies a — diversified but unitary — multimodal process of experience, at once visual, sensorimotor, and emotional.

> Contemporary neuroscience shows that what we see is not the simple "visual" recording in our brain of what stands in front of our eyes, but the result of a complex construction, whose outcome is the result of the fundamental contribution of our body with its motor potentialities, our senses and emotions, our imagination, and our memories. (Gallese 2018, 77)

As the investigation progressed, the spectrum of situations that were revealed to be able to fire up the apparatus of mirror neurons spread over a wider range of motor and sensory contingencies, each distinguished by heterogeneous scales of interference and intensity.[83] The mirror neurons selectively fire on occasions that are different from each other, but they highlight the existence of neural mechanisms that, in presiding over a particular cluster of actions, emotions, and corporeal sensations, are found to be inherently shared among all human beings. The action does not need to be caught with the eyes to set off a mirroring process; it can be experienced through other sensory channels.

> If you watch someone swinging a hammer, neural circuits in your parietal and premotor cortices become active as if you were swinging the hammer [...] These same circuits fire [...] when you simply hear someone using a hammer, which means that this empathic ability is not simply an act of visual imitation. [...] Hence, mirror neurons, in a more general way, seem to define phenomenologically our empathic relationship with the world. (Mallgrave 2013, 134)

In short, we witness episodes of neural mirroring in the following cases: 1. — when a subject observes another subject (human or animal) carry

---

83 The firing of neurons, for example, is more violent if an individual scrutinises the communication gestures of a person who is talking rather than an ape rhythmically moving its mouth to signal the lack of aggressive intentions or a dog barking (Buccino et al. 2004).

out an identical or similar motor action; 2. — when a subject recognises a depicted action, such as a static image (even when abstract and not explicitly figurative);[84] 3. — when a subject receives a communicated action, such as the sound associated with such an action or reading and listening to words describing it.[85]

The mirror neurons translate the motor scheme underlying an action, lived in the first-person or observed in others, as well as the kinetic potential multisensorially evoked by an object,[86] in a *motor programme of interaction*, namely in the motor programme requested to perform that precise gesture.

> Action implies a goal and an agent. Consequently, action recognition implies the recognition of a goal, and, from another perspective, the understanding of the agent's intentions. John sees Mary grasping an apple. By seeing her hand moving toward the apple, he recognizes what she is doing ("that's a grasp"), but also that she wants to grasp the apple, that is, her immediate, stimulus-linked "intention," or goal. (Iacoboni et al. 2005, 529)

The fundamental added value brought by mirror neurons is that they "consent to our brain to correlate the observed movements to one's own and thus to recognise the meaning" (Rizzolatti and Sinigaglia 2006, 3). Virtually enclosed within every action is a package of information articulating the overall meaning.

> An elementary gesture such as grasping a coffee cup divulges a complicated interplay of sensations (visual, tactile, olfactory, proprioceptive, etc.), motivational connections, corporeal dispositions, and motor performances that interact between themselves and with the objects around them, creating by turns more or less subtle forms of harmony. (Rizzolatti and Sinigaglia 2006, 6)

In the light of the abovementioned considerations, it is not surprising that some scientists and researchers from humanistic disciplines have hypothesised making use of these neurophysiological discoveries to

---

84 This aspect is further explored in the next section, entitled "embodied simulation."
85 In this case, we are talking about *auditory mirror neurons* (Gazzola, Aziz-Zadeh, and Keysers 2006).
86 "Object perception provides an example of embodiment which resides in the action domain. Specifically, the observation of manipulable objects triggers the same motor resources typically employed during the planning and execution of actions targeting the same objects. Hence, the motor system can also be engaged in the absence of active action execution" (Vecchiato et al. 2015).

speculate on the importance mirroring mechanisms might play in different contexts, besides the analysis of obvious functional deficits in behavioural disorders such as autism. Mirror neurons have been, for instance, examined in the interpretation of the intentions of others; in the understanding of several aspects of social cognition, language, and empathy; and, in decoding the subpersonal levels of the aesthetic experience. Vittorio Gallese, among the main figures involved in their fortuitous and fortunate discovery, suggests moving forward with "cautious optimism" (2007, 206): "mirror neurons are not 'magic cells'" (2009, 522). It mustn't be forgotten that the results of the studies conducted so far refer to profiles of cerebral triggering statistically calculated on an average of different individuals, each with a unique personal life story. "In the immediate future, neuroscientific research must focus increasingly on first-person components of the human experience and seek to understand better the personal characteristics of single subjects of experience," exhorts Gallese (2007, 203).

The idea of co-opting into the architectural investigation a possible reflection *inspired* by the principles of mirroring in actions, emotions, and corporeal sensations is so tempting and promising as to be highly seductive. It is a fact clearly intuited by Harry Francis Mallgrave, erudite expert of empathic aesthetics (Mallgrave and Ikonomou 1994), who in recent years has encouraged neuroscientific education initiatives for the architectural discipline (Mallgrave 2010, 2015b; Mallgrave and Gepshtein 2021).

> Because a building is multisensory in its myriad impressions, architecture [...] would seem to engage these neural mechanisms of mirror neurons more so than the other arts. [...] Architecture becomes the constructed means by which our embodied neural mechanisms explore and evaluate the emotional valence and affordability of our environmental fields, the embodied simulation of the materials, forms, spatial relationships, sounds, smells, tactile qualities, scales, textures, patterns, and atmosphere. (Mallgrave 2013, 139)

Embodied simulation

A strategy of enquiry, in particular, lends itself to the service of architectural research, having already been adopted in studies of an aesthetic nature (Gallese 2017b) and proving lendable, with due adaptations, to the architectural discourse:[87] the thesis of the *embodied simulation* (Gallese

---

[87] It is recognised that the architectural practice is a form of artistic expression, since it is a collector of plastic signs that carry meaning.

2005, 2019) — a process of resonance also possible with the inanimate objects that stud our architectonic surroundings, whose functional correlate is made up of mirror neurons.

Our capacity to pre-rationally make sense of the actions, emotions and sensations of others depends on embodied simulation, a functional mechanism through which the actions, emotions or sensations we see activate our own internal representations of the body states that are associated with these social stimuli, as if we were engaged in a similar action or experiencing a similar emotion or sensation. (Freedberg and Gallese 2007, 198)

This theory came into being in the early 2000s (Gallese 2003b) and, addressing the question of intersubjectivity declined as intercorporeality, it initially addressed fields of application such as linguistic understanding, psychoanalytic practice, and aesthetic experience. On the theoretical assumption that the role of embodied simulation is "that of modelling the interactions between a situated organism and its environment" (Gallese, 525), the principles it expresses can be assimilated in an architectural context. The suggestion was made by Vittorio Gallese, among the main interpreters of this model: "embodied simulation is also triggered during the experience of spatiality around our body and during the contemplation of objects [...] and is the basis of our capacity to empathize with them" (Gallese and Gattara 2015, 166). This hypothesis offers a new — experimentally demonstrable — perspective in which to probe the perceptual reactions that individuals have when they interact with a landscape of architectonic elements (not only of anthropomorphic or figurative features), evaluating the emotions that such elements evoke.[88]

A field that is now being investigated through the filter of embodied simulation is that of visual art. Vittorio Gallese and David Freedberg challenge the cognitive primacy of our reactions to the visual content of works of art (Freedberg 1989) and affirm that there are two components of the aesthetic experience involved in contemplating an artefact.

1. — the relationship between embodied empathetic feelings in the observer and the representational content of the works in terms of the actions, intentions, objects, emotions and sensations depicted in a given painting or sculpture; and
2. — the relationship between embodied empathetic feelings in the observer

---

88   "The role of embodied simulation in architectural experience becomes even more interesting if one considers emotions and sensations" (Gallese and Gattara 2015, 175).

and the quality of the work in terms of the visible traces of the artist's creative gestures, such as vigorous modeling in clay or paint, fast brushwork and signs of the movement of the hand more generally. (Freedberg and Gallese 2007, 199)

These two components (tied to the representational content of the work and to the presence of the artist, glimpsed through clear tracks of their operative actions) would always be perceptible, although in variable proportions. The theoretical intuition is reinforced thanks to a series of experiments, conducted on non-figurative abstract paintings, such as Lucio Fontana's slashed canvases (Umiltà et al. 2012) or Franz Kline's brushstrokes of colour (Sbriscia-Fioretti et al. 2013).

Despite the quality of our aesthetic fruition being influenced by our culture and the aesthetic cannons that inform it, the environment in which we were educated, the level of expertise and familiarity that we have with the work in front of us […] all these aspects, nevertheless, cannot conceal the important role carried out by our corporeal involvement in the aesthetic experience. […] To look at a painting by Kline means *also* to simulate the gestures used by the artist to make it. (Gallese 2014, 57: original italics)

The aesthetic experience is intrinsically conditioned by embodied and "universal" mechanisms of simulation (Freedberg and Gallese 2007, 197), which structure in a nonconscious and autonomous manner human reactions to the system of stimuli staged by the choreography of artefacts, designed and built by man's hand (which is, after all, the architectural context in which we live on a daily basis). "To perceive an action is equivalent to internally simulating it" (Gallese 2005, 35). The artistic origin of the sign does not affect its perception. The perceptual experience isn't influenced by the beholders' visual familiarity with the artwork or its author. There emerges only the fact that such a sign is a trace of human gestures and emotions, which can be interiorly simulated by the subject experiencing them — a subject, it is worth underlining, different (and probably distant) from whoever conceived the artwork, but united with them by a shared neural substrate. Those gestures and emotions, crystallised in the motor imprint impressed on the surface of the artefact, are animated in a process of effective co-participation and comprehension. The perceptual experience becomes viscerally incorporated and even more complete.

These concepts are further fleshed out when we speak of contact, or the involvement of the visuotactile system. A study in 2008, which planned the use of functional magnetic resonance imaging (fMRI) to examine the trigger of mirroring mechanisms at the moment that any type of tactile contact is observed, whether intentionally or accidentally, initiated both between animated agents (people) and inanimate objects (such as a chair or the branch of a plant), found that "the same mirroring/simulation principles seem to apply to the observation of any touch." To the extent that "this mechanism might underpin the activation of an abstract notion of touch" (Ebisch et al. 2008, 1621). The conclusions of the experiment are of particular importance for the architectural discipline, on the basis of the assumption that "space around us is full of objects accidentally touching each other, that is, without any animate involvement": "models of embodied simulation posit that the same neural structures involved in our own body-related experiences contribute to the conceptualization of what we observe in the world around us" (Ebisch et al., 1621). In other words, it seems that human beings can interiorly simulate the tactile values of inert elements that make up their environment.

In a Nutshell

Intuiting the meaning of the architectural experience is perhaps one of the greatest challenges the discipline can undertake. As the American philosopher Mark Johnson explains, "architecture is our most human (and potentially humane) way of relating to our environing world." It "is an act of imaginative problem solving that resonates with the deepest levels of our connection to our environment" (2002, 86; 88).

In every science, there are aspects that we understand, or at least believe we do, and others that we would like to understand better. Alas, the two do not always coincide, although overlapping to some extent. Opportunities to comprehend often emerge in unexpected places, from issues that initially have scarce applied interest. The scientific exploration of the architectural experience is no exception, in perennial equilibrium between two focal points: "on the one hand, we have the need for something stable and universal — a basis for prediction and recognition — and, on the other, the need for personal and emotional identification" (Thiis-Evensen 1987, 8).

The atmospheric dimension — or rather, the quintessence of the vague and ephemeral, intimate and emotional, apparently not concrete nor practical — offers an original theoretical horizon to investigate the experiential basis that sustains architectural activity.

The journey through the universe of atmospheric sensibility undertaken in this book had the merit (or, at least, this is the hope) of setting, within the architectural discipline, a perimeter around the field of existence of the impalpable atmospheric dynamics. To understand (a bit better) the entity of the atmospheric phenomenon was the first step to finding a congruent manner of attempting to identify and ascribe it in a formal sense system. The idea of seeking a definition for a construct, up to now entrusted to poetic allusion, by trespassing on the scientific domain, proved an interesting strategy — at the very least to empty the concept of a series of clichés. First of all, the one stating that atmosphere "by definition [...] lacks definition" (Wigley 1998a, 27). This widely accepted status of vagueness has of course served its seductive expressive power, but the affirmation of a shared semantic substrate seemed necessary from the start, in order to take the research forward. With the proposed definition (namely: *atmosphere as a state of emotional resonance and potential consonance between the perceiving subject and their architectonically arranged environment*), the semantic core of the atmospheric root was improved on, consolidating the area of atmospheric study as a scenario of autonomous enquiry — here formalized for the architectural discipline as completely and knowingly as possible.

The atmospheric enigma has not been solved. Some order has been imposed. After all, atmospheres are still "one of the most complex aspects tackled in architecture," being "that bit of air that remains when you take away the walls, floor, and ceiling."[1] This, in its genuine essentiality, is the fundamental lesson I treasure from the nature of atmospheres, and the first I received. It was given to me by Antonio, master of atmospheres, to whom this journey is dedicated.[2]

---

1 Antonio Jiménez Torrecillas, interviewed in the video-documentary *Spain Alight* (minute 16:10), directed by Jorge Cosmen and available online at Vimeo (www.vimeo.com/29795661, last accessed 11 December 2021) © 2011 Narita Estudio / Stone Designs / Les Films Anonymes.
2 Antonio Jiménez Torrecillas (Hellín, 1962 — Granada, 2015). For a tribute, see Canepa 2020.

Bibliography

Notes

Quotations cited from the original; no English-language sources have been translated by the translator.

Ábalos, Iñaki, and Sentkiewicz, Renata. 2015. *Essays on Thermodynamics, Architecture and Beauty*. Barcelona and New York, NY: Actar.

Achleitner, Friedrich. 1997. "Ritorno al moderno? L'architettura di Peter Zumthor." *Casabella* 648, year LXI, 9: 52–55.

Adcock, Craig. 1990. *James Turrell: The Art of Light and Space*. Berkeley, CA and Oxford: University of California (UC) Press.

Albini, Franco. 2005. "Le mie esperienze di architetto nelle esposizioni in Italia e all'estero / My Experiences as an Architect in Exhibitions in Italy and Abroad" (1954). *Casabella* 730, year LXIX, 2: 9–12; 99–100.

Albright, Thomas D., Jessell, Thomas M., Kandel, Eric R., and Posner, Michael I. 2000. "Neural Science: A Century of Progress and the Mysteries that Remain." *Cell/Neuron* 100, 25 (Millennial Review Supplement): s1–s55. DOI: 10.1016/s0896-6273(00)80912-5.

Andersen, Michael A. 2012. "In Conversation: Peter Zumthor and Juhani Pallasmaa." *AD Architectural Design* 82, 6 (Human Experience and Place: Sustaining Identity): 22–25. DOI: 10.1002/ad.1487.

Anderson, Ben. 2009. "Affective Atmospheres." *Emotion, Space and Society* 2, 2: 77–81. DOI: 10.1016/j.emospa.2009.08.005.

Anderson, Ben. 2014. *Encountering Affect: Capacities, Apparatuses, Conditions*. Farnham and Burlington, VT: Ashgate.

Ando, Tadao. 2021. "Confrontarsi con la natura / Confronting Nature." *Domus* 1056: 1 (editorial).

Asu Schroer, Sara, and Schmitt, Susanne B. (eds.). 2018. *Exploring Atmospheres Ethnographically*. Anthropological Studies of Creativity and Perception. Abingdon and New York, NY: Routledge.

Augustin, Sally. 2009. *Place Advantage: Applied Psychology for Interior Architecture*. Hoboken, NJ: Wiley.

Augustin, Sally. 2017. "Designing for Humans: The Essentials." In *Conscious Cities: Bridging Neuroscience, Architecture and Technology — An Anthology*, vol. II, ed. by A. Fritz and I. Palti, 60–63. London: Conscious Cities, The Centric Lab.

Augustin, Sally, and Coleman, Cindy. 2012. *The Designer's Guide to Doing Research: Applying Knowledge to Inform Design*. Hoboken, NJ: Wiley.

Bachelard, Gaston. 1971. *The Poetics of Reverie: Childhood, Language, and the Cosmos* (1960). Trans. by D. Russell. Boston, MA: Beacon Press.

Bachelard, Gaston. 1994. *The Poetics of Space* (1958). Trans. by M. Jolas. Boston, MA: Beacon Press.

Baglione, Chiara. 2006. "Costruire col fuoco: La cappella nell'Eifel — Chiara Baglione intervista Peter Zumthor / Interview with Peter Zumthor." *Casabella* 747, year LXX, 9: 65–67; 91–92.

Baglione, Chiara. 2007. "Nel silenzio / In the Silence." *Casabella* 758, year LXXI, 9: 144–153; 163.

Banham, Reyner. 1965. "A Home is Not a House." Illustrated by F. Dallegret. *Art in America* 53, 2: 70–79.

Banham, Reyner. 1969. *The Architecture of the Well-Tempered Environment*. London: The Architectural Press — Chicago, IL: The University of Chicago Press.

Barrett, Lisa F., Mesquita, Batja, Ochsner, Kevin N., and Gross, James J. 2007. "The Experience of Emotion." *Annual Review of Psychology* 58, 1: 373–403. DOI: 10.1146/annurev.psych.58.110405.085709.

Baudrillard, Jean. 1996. *The System of Objects* (1968). Trans. by J. Benedict. London and New York, NY: Verso.

Baudrillard, Jean, and Nouvel, Jean. 2002. *The Singular Objects of Architecture* (2000). Trans. by R. Bononno. Minneapolis, MN and London: University of Minnesota Press.

Bell, Lynne, Vogt, Julia, Willemse, Cesco, Routledge, Tim, Butler, Laurie T., and Sakaki, Michiko. 2018. "Beyond Self-Report: A Review of Physiological and Neuroscientific Methods to Investigate Consumer Behavior." *Frontiers in Psychology* 9: 1655, 1–16. DOI: 10.3389/fpsyg.2018.01655.

Benedito, Silvia. 2013. "On Atmospheres and Design." Syllabus, Harvard University, Graduate School of Design (GSD), Landscape Department, ADV 09128 Seminar (spring term).

Benedito, Silvia. 2021. *Atmosphere Anatomies: On Design, Weather, and Sensation*. Baden: Lars Müller.

Benjamin, Walter. 2007. "The Work of Art in the Age of Mechanical Reproduction." In *Illuminations: Essays and Reflections* (1968), ed. by H. Arendt and trans. by H. Zohn, 217–251. New York, NY: Schocken Books. The original source of the essay published in this collection is "L'œuvre d'art à l'époque de sa reproduction mécanisée" (1936). *Zeitschrift für Sozialforschung* 5, 1: 40–68. DOI: 10.5840/zfs193651130.

Bermúdez, José L. 2020. *Cognitive Science: An Introduction to the Science of the Mind* (2010). 3rd edn. Cambridge and New York, NY: Cambridge University Press (CUP).

Bibliography

Bessoudo, Mark. 2017. "Health, Wellness, and Experience in the Built Environment: From Green Buildings to Conscious Cities." In *Conscious Cities: Bridging Neuroscience, Architecture and Technology — An Anthology*, vol. II, ed. by A. Fritz and I. Palti, 76–83. London: Conscious Cities, The Centric Lab.

Bille, Mikkel, Bjerregaard, Peter, and Sørensen, Tim F. 2015. "Staging Atmospheres: Materiality, Culture, and the Texture of the In-Between." *Emotion, Space and Society* 15 (Staging Atmospheres): 31–38. DOI: 10.1016/j.emospa.2014.11.002.

Bloomer, Kent C., and Moore, Charles W., with a contribution by R.J. Yudell. 1977. *Body, Memory, and Architecture*. New Haven, CT and London: Yale University Press (YUP).

Boella, Laura. 2006. *Sentire l'altro: Conoscere e praticare l'empatia*. Minima, 82. Milano: Raffaello Cortina.

Böhme, Gernot. 1991. "Über Synästhesien / On Synaesthesiae." *Daidalos. Architektur Kunst Kultur / Architecture Art Culture* 41 (Provokation der Sinne / Provocation of the Senses): 26–37.

Böhme, Gernot. 1993. "Atmosphere as the Fundamental Concept of a New Aesthetics." *Thesis Eleven* 36, 1: 113–126. DOI: 10.1177/072551369303600107.

Böhme, Gernot. 1995a. *Atmosphäre: Essays zur neuen Ästhetik*. Frankfurt am Main: Suhrkamp.

Böhme, Gernot. 1995b. "Inszenierte Materialität / Staged Materiality." *Daidalos. Architektur Kunst Kultur / Architecture Art Culture* 56 (Magie der Werkstoffe / Magic of Materials): 36–43.

Böhme, Gernot. 1998. "Atmosphäre als Begriff der Ästhetik / Atmosphere as an Aesthetic Concept." *Daidalos. Architektur Kunst Kultur / Architecture Art Culture* 68 (Konstruktion von Atmosphären / Constructing Atmospheres): 112–115.

Böhme, Gernot. 2001. *Aisthetik: Vorlesungen über Ästhetik als allgemeine Wahrnehmungslehre*. München: Wilhelm Fink.

Böhme, Gernot. 2005. "Atmosphere as the Subject Matter of Architecture." In *Herzog and de Meuron: Natural History*, ed. by P. Ursprung, 398–406. Baden: Lars Müller.

Böhme, Gernot. 2006. *Architektur und Atmosphäre*. München: Wilhelm Fink.

Böhme, Gernot. 2013a. "Metaphors in Architecture — a Metaphor?" In *Metaphors in Architecture and Urbanism: An Introduction*, ed. by A. Gerber and B. Patterson, 47–58. Architekturen, 19. Bielefeld: Transcript.

Böhme, Gernot. 2013b. "Atmosphere as Mindful Physical Presence in Space / Sfeer als bewuste fysieke aanwezigheid in de ruimte" (2006). *OASE. Journal for Architecture / Tijdschrift voor architectuur* 91 (Building Atmosphere / Sfeer bouwen): 21–32.

Böhme, Gernot. 2013c. "Synaesthesiae within the Scope of a Phenomenology of Perception" (2002). *Wolkenkuckucksheim | Cloud-Cuckoo-Land | Воздушный замок (W|C|B). International Journal of Architectural Theory* 18, 31 (Synaesthesia. Body — Space / Architecture): 23–33.

Böhme, Gernot. 2013d. "Encountering Atmospheres: A Reflection on the Concept of Atmosphere in the Work of Juhani Pallasmaa and Peter Zumthor / Een treffen van sferen: Reflectie op het begrip sfeer bij Juhani Pallasmaa en Peter Zumthor." *OASE.*

Journal for Architecture / Tijdschrift voor architectuur 91 (Building Atmosphere / Sfeer bouwen): 93–100.

Böhme, Gernot. 2013e. "The Art of the Stage Set as a Paradigm for an Aesthetics of Atmospheres." *Ambiances. International Journal of Sensory Environment, Architecture and Urban Space*, Rediscovering: n.p. DOI: 10.4000/ambiances.315.

Böhme, Gernot. 2014. "Atmospheres: New Perspectives for Architecture and Design." In P. Tidwell (ed.), 2014, 7–14.

Böhme, Gernot. 2017a. *Critique of Aesthetic Capitalism*. Atmospheric Spaces, 1. Milano and Udine: Mimesis International.

Böhme, Gernot. 2017b. *Atmospheric Architectures: The Aesthetics of Felt Spaces* (2006). Ed. and trans. by A.C. Engels-Schwarzpaul. London and New York, NY: Bloomsbury.

Böhme, Gernot. 2017c. *The Aesthetics of Atmospheres*. Ed. by J.P. Thibaud. Ambiances, Atmospheres and Sensory Experiences of Space, 1. Abingdon and New York, NY: Routledge.

Bollnow, Otto F. 1941. *Das Wesen der Stimmungen*. Frankfurt am Main: Vittorio Klostermann.

Bollnow, Otto F. 2020. *Human Space* (1963). Trans. by C. Shuttleworth. Atmospheric Spaces, 8. Milano and Udine: Mimesis International.

Borch, Christian (ed.). 2014. *Architectural Atmospheres: On the Experience and Politics of Architecture*. Basel: Birkhäuser.

Bower, Isabella, Tucker, Richard, and Enticott, Peter G. 2019. "Impact of Built Environment Design on Emotion Measured via Neurophysiological Correlates and Subjective Indicators: A Systematic Review." *Journal of Environmental Psychology* 66: 101344, 1–11. DOI: 10.1016/j.jenvp.2019.101344.

Brennan, Teresa. 2004. *The Transmission of Affect*. Ithaca, NY and London: Cornell University Press.

Bruno, Giuliana. 2002. *Atlas of Emotion: Journeys in Art, Architecture, and Film*. London and New York, NY: Verso.

Bucci, Marco. 2005. "L'arte del porgere: Franco Albini e l'architettura delle esposizioni / The Art of Offering: Franco Albini and the Architecture of Exhibitions." *Casabella* 730, year LXIX, 2: 13–15; 100–101.

Buccino, Giovanni, Binkofski, Ferdinand, and Riggio, Lucia. 2004. "The Mirror Neuron System and Action Recognition." *Brain and Language* 89, 2: 370–376. DOI: 10.1016/S0093-934X(03)00356-0.

Buccino, Giovanni, Lui, Fausta, Canessa, Nicola, Patteri, Ilaria, Lagravinese, Giovanna, Benuzzi, Francesca, Porro, Carlo A., and Rizzolatti, Giacomo. 2004. "Neural Circuits Involved in the Recognition of Actions Performed by Nonconspecifics: An fMRI Study." *Journal of Cognitive Neuroscience* 16, 1: 114–126. DOI: 10.1162/089892904322755601.

Buchert, Margitta. 2021. "Design Knowledges on the Move." In *The Tacit Dimension: Architecture Knowledge and Scientific Research*, ed. by L. Schrijver, 83–96. Leuven: Leuven University Press (LUP). DOI: 10.2307/j.ctv1mgm7ng.8.

Buiatti, Eleonora. 2014. *Forma Mentis: Neuroergonomia sensoriale applicata alla progettazione*. Milano: FrancoAngeli.

Bibliography

Canepa, Elisabetta. 2017. "Contro la tirannia dell'occhio." In *Ordinary Rooms*, ed. by E. Canepa, 9–16. History of the Future, 1. Genova: Sagep editori.

Canepa, Elisabetta. 2018. "A discolpa delle archistar©." *Pièra. Magazine of Treviso Association of Architects* 7 (Gli anni duemila): 88–93.

Canepa, Elisabetta. 2019. "Neurocosmi: La dimensione atmosferica tra architettura e neuroscienze." Doctoral dissertation, University of Genoa. Institutional Research Information System (IRIS): http://hdl.handle.net/11567/944826.

Canepa, Elisabetta. 2020. "L'Architettura Bella. Due lezioni di Antonio Jiménez Torrecillas." *GUD. A Magazine about Architecture, Design and Cities* 2 (Conclusus): 36–47.

Canepa, Elisabetta. 2021. "Fenomenografia atmosferica: Ovvero, la strategia del procedere per gradi di intimità." In *Un anno di didattica: Innovazione e ricerca nella scuola di architettura di Genova*, 15–19; 130–131. Opera metrica, 4. Genova: Sagep editori.

Canepa, Elisabetta, Avanzino, Laura, Fassio, Anna, Lagravinese, Giovanna, and Scelsi, Valter. 2018. "Neurocosmos: The Emotional and Cognitive Correlates of Architectural Atmospheres." In *ANFA 2018 Conference — "Shared Behavioral Outcomes:" Abstracts Volume*, ed. by the Academy of Neuroscience for Architecture (ANFA), 40–41. San Diego, CA: 20–22 September 2018.

Canepa, Elisabetta, Scelsi, Valter, Fassio, Anna, Avanzino, Laura, Lagravinese, Giovanna, and Chiorri, Carlo. 2019. "Atmospheres: Feeling Architecture by Emotions. Preliminary Neuroscientific Insights on Atmospheric Perception in Architecture." *Ambiances. International Journal of Sensory Environment, Architecture and Urban Space* 5 (Phenomenographies: Describing Urban and Architectural Atmospheres): n.p. DOI: 10.4000/ambiances.2907.

Carnevali, Barbara. 2006. "'Aura' e 'ambiance': Léon Daudet tra Proust e Benjamin." *Rivista di estetica* 33, year XLVI, 3 (Atmosfere): 117–141.

Carney, James. 2020. "Thinking Avant la Lettre: A Review of 4E Cognition." *Evolutionary Studies in Imaginative Culture* 4, 1 (Symposium on Meaning and Evolution): 77–90. DOI: 10.26613/esic/4.1.172.

Casciani, Stefano. 2007. "Il Santo e l'Architetto / A Saint and an Architect." *Domus* 906: 52–59.

Chatterjee, Anjan, and Vartanian, Oshin. 2014. "Neuroaesthetics." *Trends in Cognitive Sciences* 18, 7: 370–375. DOI: 10.1016/j.tics.2014.03.003.

Condia, Robert J. (ed.). 2020a. *Meaning in Architecture: Affordances, Atmosphere and Mood*. Manhattan, KS: New Prairie Press.

Condia, Robert J. (ed.). 2020b. *Affordances and the Potential for Architecture*. Manhattan, KS: New Prairie Press.

Condia, Robert J. 2021. "Architecture as Manifest Action, Experience, and Atmosphere." Syllabus, Kansas State University, College of Architecture, Planning and Design (APDesign), Architecture Department, ADS7 Interdisciplinary Studio (fall term).

Condia, Robert J., and Luczak, Michael. 2014. "On Mood and Aesthetic Experience in Architecture." In *ANFA 2014 Conference: Presenter Abstracts*, ed. by the Academy of Neuroscience for Architecture (ANFA), 24–25. San Diego, CA: 18–20 September 2014.

Connor, Steven. 2010. *The Matter of Air: Science and the Art of the Ethereal*. London: Reaktion Books.

Constant. 1998. "New Babylon — Ten Years On" (1980). Trans. by R. de Jong-Dalziel. In M. Wigley (ed.), 1998b, 232–236.

Coole, Diana, and Frost, Samantha (eds.). 2010. *New Materialisms: Ontology, Agency, and Politics*. Durham, NC and London: Duke University Press (DUP).

Corbin, Alain. 1986. *The Foul and the Fragrant: Odor and the French Social Imagination* (1982). Leamington Spa, Hamburg, and New York, NY: Berg.

Coss, Richard G. 2003. "The Role of Evolved Perceptual Biases in Art and Design." In *Evolutionary Aesthetics*, ed. by E. Voland and K. Grammer, 69–130. Berlin and Heidelberg: Springer. DOI: 10.1007/978-3-662-07142-7_4.

Croce, Benedetto. 1967. "L'estetica della 'Einfühlung'" (1934). In *Storia dell'estetica per saggi*, 239–246. Roma and Bari: Laterza.

Cuff, Benjamin M.P., Brown, Sarah J., Taylor, Laura, and Howat, Douglas J. 2016. "Empathy: A Review of the Concept" (2014). *Emotion Review* 8, 2: 144–153. DOI: 10.1177/1754073914558466.

Curtis, Robin, and Elliott, Richard G. (trans.). 2014. "An Introduction to *Einfühlung*." *Art in Translation* 6, 4: 353–376. DOI: 10.1080/17561310.2014.11425535.

Damasio, Antonio R. 1994. *Descartes' Error: Emotion, Reason, and the Human Brain*. New York, NY: Avon Books.

De Freitas, Elizabeth, and Rousell, David. 2021. "Atmospheric Intensities: Skin Conductance and the Collective Sensing Body." In *Affects, Interfaces, Events*, ed. by B.M. Stavning Thomsen, J. Kofoed, and J. Fritsch, 221–241. Lancaster, PA and Vancouver: Imbricate! Press.

De Matteis, Federico. 2020. "Atmosphere in Architecture." In *International Lexicon of Aesthetics* (ILAe). Spring edn. Sesto San Giovanni: Mimesis. DOI: 10.7413/18258630074.

De Matteis, Federico. 2021. *Affective Spaces: Architecture and the Living Body*. Ambiances, Atmospheres and Sensory Experiences of Spaces, 8. Abingdon and New York, NY: Routledge.

De Matteis, Federico, Bille, Mikkel, Griffero, Tonino, and Jelić, Andrea. 2019. "Phenomenographies: Describing the Plurality of Atmospheric Worlds." *Ambiances. International Journal of Sensory Environment, Architecture and Urban Space* 5 (Phenomenographies: Describing Urban and Architectural Atmospheres): n.p. DOI: 10.4000/ambiances.2526.

De Rosa, Agostino (ed.). 2007. *James Turrell: Geometrie di Luce. Roden Crater Project*. Milano: Mondadori Electa.

Debord, Guy-Ernest (ed.). 1958. *Internationale situationniste* 1. Paris.

Debord, Guy-Ernest. 2002. "Report on the Construction of Situations and on the Terms of Organization and Action of the International Situationist Tendency" (1957). In *Guy Debord and the Situationist International: Texts and Documents*, ed. and trans. by T. McDonough, 29–50. Cambridge, MA and London: The MIT Press.

Décosterd, Jean-Gilles, and Rahm, Philippe. 2002. *Physiological Architecture / Architecture physiologique*. Basel, Berlin, and Boston, MA: Birkhäuser.

Deleuze, Gilles, and Guattari, Félix. 1987. *A Thousand Plateaus: Capitalism and Schizophrenia* (1980). Trans. by B. Massumi. Minneapolis, MN and London: University of Minnesota Press.

Delplanque, Sylvain, and Sander, David. 2021. "A Fascinating but Risky Case of Reverse Inference: From Measures to Emotions!" *Food Quality and Preference* 92: 104183, 1–5. DOI: 10.1016/j.foodqual.2021.104183.

Di Dio, Cinzia, and Gallese, Vittorio. 2009. "Neuroaesthetics: A Review." *Current Opinion in Neurobiology* 19, 6: 682–687. DOI: 10.1016/j.conb.2009.09.001.

Di Pellegrino, Giuseppe, Fadiga, Luciano, Fogassi, Leonardo, Gallese, Vittorio, and Rizzolatti, Giacomo. 1992. "Understanding Motor Events: A Neurophysiological Study." *Experimental Brain Research* 91, 1: 176–180. DOI: 10.1007/BF00230027.

Di Pellegrino, Giuseppe, and Làdavas, Elisabetta. 2015. "Peripersonal Space in the Brain." *Neuropsychologia. An International Journal in Behavioural and Cognitive Neuroscience* 66: 126–133. DOI: 10.1016/j.neuropsychologia.2014.11.011.

Di Stefano, Elisabetta. 2012. *Hyperaesthetics: Art, Nature, Everyday Life, and New Technologies*. Aesthetica Preprint, 95. Palermo: International Centre for the Study of Aesthetics.

Durisch, Thomas (ed.). 2014. *Peter Zumthor. 1985–2013: Buildings and Projects*. Zürich: Scheidegger und Spiess.

Ebisch, Sjoerd J.H., Perrucci, Mauro G., Ferretti, Antonio, Del Gratta, Cosimo, Romani, Gian Luca, and Gallese, Vittorio. 2008. "The Sense of Touch: Embodied Simulation in a Visuotactile Mirroring Mechanism for Observed Animate or Inanimate Touch." *Journal of Cognitive Neuroscience* 20, 9: 1611–1623. DOI: 10.1162/jocn.2008.20111.

Edensor, Tim, and Sumartojo, Shanti. 2015. "Designing Atmospheres: Introduction to Special Issue." *Visual Communication* 14, 3 (Designing Atmospheres): 251–265. DOI: 10.1177/1470357215582305.

Eisenman, Peter. 1992. "Oltre lo sguardo: L'architettura nell'epoca dei media elettronici / Visions' Unfolding: Architecture in the Age of Electronic Media." *Domus* 734: 19–24.

Eliasson, Olafur. 2010. *Olafur Eliasson: Your Chance Encounter*. Baden: Lars Müller.

Eliasson, Olafur. 2012. *Never Tired of Looking at Each Other — Only the Mountain and I*. Beijing: The Pavilion.

Eliasson, Olafur. 2016. *Studio Olafur Eliasson: Unspoken Spaces*. London: Thames and Hudson (T&H).

Eliasson, Olafur. 2018. "Conoscere Sentire Agire." *Intertwining* 1 (Unfolding Art and Science): 56–57.

Endell, August. 1995. *Vom Sehen: Texte 1896–1925. Über Architektur, Formkunst und "Die Schönheit der großen Stadt."* Ed. by H. David. Basel, Berlin, and Boston, MA: Birkhäuser.

Endell, August. 2018. *The Beauty of the Metropolis* (1908). Trans. by J.J. Conway. Berlin: Rixdorf Editions.

Espuelas, Fernando. 1999. *El claro en el bosque: Reflexiones sobre el vacío en arquitectura*. Barcelona: Fundación Caja de Arquitectos.

Ferrari, Pier Francesco, and Rizzolatti, Giacomo. 2014. "Mirror Neuron Research: The Past and the Future." *Philosophical Transactions of the Royal Society B. Biological Sciences* 369, 1644: 20130169, 1–4. DOI: 10.1098/rstb.2013.0169.

Fitzgerald, Des, and Callard, Felicity. 2014. "Social Science and Neuroscience beyond Interdisciplinarity: Experimental Entanglements." *Theory, Culture and Society* 32, 1: 3–32. DOI: 10.1177/0263276414537319.

Ford, Thomas H. 2018. *Wordsworth and the Poetics of Air: Atmospheric Romanticism in a Time of Climate Change*. Cambridge and New York, NY: Cambridge University Press (CUP).

Forty, Adrian. 2000. *Words and Buildings: A Vocabulary of Modern Architecture*. New York, NY: Thames and Hudson (T&H).

Frampton, Kenneth. 1995. "Introduction: Reflections on the Scope of the Tectonic." In *Studies in Tectonic Culture: The Poetics of Construction in Nineteenth and Twentieth Century Architecture*, ed. by J. Cava, 1–27. Cambridge, MA and London: The MIT Press — Chicago, IL: Graham Foundation for Advanced Studies in the Fine Arts.

Freedberg, David. 1989. *The Power of Images: Studies in the History and Theory of Response*. Chicago, IL: The University of Chicago Press (UCP).

Freedberg, David, and Gallese, Vittorio. 2007. "Motion, Emotion and Empathy in Esthetic Experience." *Trends in Cognitive Sciences* 11, 5: 197–203. DOI: 10.1016/j.tics.2007.02.003.

Frichot, Hélène. 2008. "Olafur Eliasson and the Circulation of Affects and Percepts: In Conversation." *AD. Architectural Design* 78, 3 (Interior Atmospheres): 30–35. DOI: 10.1002/ad.671.

Fujimoto, Sou. 2010. "Futuro Primitivo / Primitive Future." *El Croquis* 151 (Sou Fujimoto: 2003/2010): 198–214.

Fuller, R. Buckminster. 1969. *Operating Manual for Spaceship Earth*. Touchstone Books. New York, NY: Simon and Schuster — Carbondale, IL: Southern Illinois University (SIU) Press.

Gabrieli, John D.E., Ghosh, Satrajit S., and Whitfield-Gabrieli, Susan. 2015. "Prediction as a Humanitarian and Pragmatic Contribution from Human Cognitive Neuroscience." *Neuron* 85, 1: 11–26. DOI: 10.1016/j.neuron.2014.10.047.

Gallese, Vittorio. 2003a. "The Roots of Empathy: The Shared Manifold Hypothesis and the Neural Basis of Intersubjectivity." *Psychopathology* 36: 171–180. DOI: 10.1159/000072786.

Gallese, Vittorio. 2003b. "The Manifold Nature of Interpersonal Relations: The Quest for a Common Mechanism." *Philosophical Transactions of the Royal Society B. Biological Sciences* 358, 1431: 517–528. DOI: 10.1098/rstb.2002.1234.

Gallese, Vittorio. 2005. "Embodied Simulation: From Neurons to Phenomenal Experience." *Phenomenology and the Cognitive Sciences* 4: 23–48. DOI: 10.1007/s11097-005-4737-z.

Gallese, Vittorio. 2006. "Corpo vivo, simulazione incarnata e intersoggettività: Una prospettiva neurofenomenologica." In *Neurofenomenologia: Le scienze della mente e la sfida dell'esperienza cosciente*, ed. by M. Cappuccio, 293–326. Milano: Bruno Mondadori.

Gallese, Vittorio. 2007. "Dai neuroni specchio alla consonanza intenzionale: Meccanismi neurofisiologici dell'intersoggettività." *Rivista di Psicoanalisi* 53, 1: 197–208.

Gallese, Vittorio. 2009. "Mirror Neurons, Embodied Simulation, and the Neural Basis of Social Identification." *Psychoanalytic Dialogues* 19, 5: 519–536. DOI: 10.1080/10481880903231910.

Gallese, Vittorio. 2014. "Arte, corpo, cervello: Per un'estetica sperimentale." *Micromega* 2: 49–67.

Gallese, Vittorio. 2015. "L'architettura della conoscenza secondo Harry Mallgrave." Foreword to H.F. Mallgrave, *L'empatia degli spazi: Architettura e neuroscienze* (2013), IX–XVIII. Italian edn. Milano: Raffaello Cortina.

Gallese, Vittorio. 2017a. "Visions of the Body: Embodied Simulation and Aesthetic Experience." *Aisthesis. Pratiche, linguaggi e saperi dell'estetico* 10, 1 (Ways of Imitation): 41–50. DOI: 10.13128/Aisthesis-20902.

Gallese, Vittorio. 2017b. "The Empathic Body in Experimental Aesthetics: Embodied Simulation and Art." In *Empathy: Epistemic Problems and Cultural-Historical Perspectives of a Cross-Disciplinary Concept*, ed. by V. Lux and S. Weigel, 181–199. Palgrave Studies in the Theory and History of Psychology. London: Palgrave Macmillan. DOI: 10.1057/978-1-137-51299-4_7.

Gallese, Vittorio. 2018. "The Problem of Images: A View from the Brain-Body." *Phenomenology and Mind* 14 (Perception and Aesthetic Experience): 70–79. DOI: 10.13128/Phe_Mi-23626.

Gallese, Vittorio. 2019. "Embodied Simulation: Its Bearing on Aesthetic Experience and the Dialogue Between Neuroscience and the Humanities." *Gestalt Theory. An International Multidisciplinary Journal* 41, 2 (What is What? Focus on Transdisciplinary Concepts and Terminology in Neuroaesthetics, Cognition and Poetics): 113–127. DOI: 10.2478/gth-2019-0013.

Gallese, Vittorio, and Cuccio, Valentina. 2015. "The Paradigmatic Body: Embodied Simulation, Intersubjectivity, the Bodily Self, and Language." *Open MIND*, ed. by T. Metzinger and J.M. Windt, 14 (T): 1–22. Frankfurt am Main: MIND Group. DOI: 10.15502/9783958570269.

Gallese, Vittorio, and Gattara, Alessandro. 2015. "Embodied Simulation, Aesthetics, and Architecture: An Experimental Aesthetic Approach." In *Mind in Architecture: Neuroscience, Embodiment, and the Future of Design*, ed. by S. Robinson and J. Pallasmaa, 161–179. Cambridge, MA and London: The MIT Press. Stable URL: http://www.jstor.org/stable/j.ctt17kk8bm.12.

Gallese, Vittorio, and Lakoff, George. 2005. "The Brain's Concepts: The Role of the Sensory-Motor System in Conceptual Knowledge." *Cognitive Neuropsychology* 22, 3/4: 455–479. DOI: 10.1080/02643290442000310.

Gallese, Vittorio, and Sinigaglia, Corrado. 2011. "What Is So Special about Embodied Simulation?" *Trends in Cognitive Sciences* 15, 11: 512–519. DOI: 10.1016/j.tics.2011.09.003.

Gandy, Matthew. 2017. "Urban Atmospheres." *Cultural Geographies* 24, 3: 353–374. DOI: 10.1177/1474474017712995.

Gardner, Howard. 1985. *The Mind's New Science: A History of the Cognitive Revolution*. New York, NY: Basic Books.

Gardner, Howard. 1999. *Intelligence Reframed: Multiple Intelligences for the 21st Century*. New York, NY: Basic Books.

Gazzola, Valeria, Aziz-Zadeh, Lisa, and Keysers, Christian. 2006. "Empathy and the Somatotopic Auditory Mirror System in Humans." *Current Biology* 16, 18: 1824–1829. DOI: 10.1016/j.cub.2006.07.072.

Giberti, Massimiliano. 2012. *Piccolo Manuale d'Uso per l'Architettura Contemporanea*. Milano: 22 Publishing.

Giedion, Sigfried. 1954. *Space, Time and Architecture: The Growth of a New Tradition* (1941). 3rd edn, enlarged version. Cambridge, MA: Harvard University Press (HUP).

Govan, Michael, and Kim, Christine Y. 2013. *James Turrell: A Retrospective*. Los Angeles, CA: Los Angeles County Museum of Art (LACMA) — New York, NY: DelMonico Books.

Gregory, Paola. 2020. "Atmosfera." In *Enciclopedia Italiana di Scienze, Lettere ed Arti*. 10th Appendix (Parole del XXI secolo), 115–119. Roma: Istituto della Enciclopedia Italiana Treccani.

Griffero, Tonino. 2005a. "Corpi e atmosfere: Il 'punto di vista' delle cose." In *Il luogo dello spettatore: Forme dello sguardo nella cultura delle immagini*, ed. by A. Somaini, 283–318. Milano: Vita e Pensiero (V&P).

Griffero, Tonino. 2005b. "Non dentro ma fuori: Le atmosfere come spazi emozionali." *Oltreconfine. Annuario della Società Filosofica Feronia — Società Filosofica Italiana (SFI) di Latina*, 12–17.

Griffero, Tonino. 2010. "Atmosfere: Non metafore ma quasi-cose." In *Metafore del vivente: Linguaggi e ricerca scientifica tra filosofia, bios e psiche*, ed. by E. Gagliasso and G. Frezza, 123–131. Milano: FrancoAngeli.

Griffero, Tonino. 2012. *Storia dell'estetica moderna*. Crossroads: Filosofia e Scienze Sociali, 1. Roma: Edizioni Nuova Cultura.

Griffero, Tonino. 2013. "The Atmospheric 'Skin' of the City." *Ambiances. International Journal of Sensory Environment, Architecture and Urban Space*, Varia: n.p. DOI: 10.4000/ambiances.399.

Griffero, Tonino. 2014a. *Atmospheres: Aesthetics of Emotional Spaces* (2010). Trans. by S. de Sanctis. Farnham and Burlington, VT: Ashgate.

Griffero, Tonino. 2014b. "Atmospheres and Lived Space." *Studia Phænomenologica. The Journal of the Romanian Society for Phenomenology* 14 (Place, Environment, Atmosphere): 29–51. DOI: 10.5840/studphaen2014144.

Griffero, Tonino. 2014c. "Architectural Affordances: The Atmospheric Authority of Spaces." In P. Tidwell (ed.), 2014, 15–47.

Griffero, Tonino. 2014d. "Estetica patica: Appunti per un'atmosferologia neofenomenologica." *Studi di estetica. Italian Journal of Aesthetics*, year XLII, series IV, 1–2 (Tra il sensibile e le arti: Trent'anni di estetica): 161–183.

Griffero, Tonino. 2015. "Trovato o creato? Il *genius loci* come esperienza (atmosferica)." In *Sensibilia 9: Genius Loci*, ed. by S. Pedone and M. Tedeschini, 155–181. Sesto San Giovanni: Mimesis.

Griffero, Tonino. 2019. "Is There Such a Thing as an 'Atmospheric Turn'? Instead of an Introduction." In *Atmosphere and Aesthetics: A Plural Perspective*, ed. by T. Griffero and M. Tedeschini, 11–62. Cham: Palgrave Macmillan.

Griffero, Tonino. 2020a. *Places, Affordances, Atmospheres: A Pathic Aesthetics*. Ambiances, Atmospheres and Sensory Experiences of Spaces, 3. Abingdon and New York, NY: Routledge.

Griffero, Tonino. 2020b. "Better to Be in Tune: Between Resonance and Responsivity." *Studi di Estetica. Italian Journal of Aesthetics*, year XLVIII, series IV, 2 (Sensibilia 13: Resonance): 93–118. DOI: 10.7413/18258646128.

Griffero, Tonino. 2020c. "Where Do We Stand on Atmospheres?" In *Resounding Spaces: Approaching Musical Atmospheres*, ed. by F. Scassillo, 11–24. Atmospheric Spaces, 7. Milano and Udine: Mimesis International.

Griffero, Tonino. 2020d. "Otto Friedrich Bollnow and Lived Space." In O.F. Bollnow, 2020, 13–27.

Griffero, Tonino, and Moretti, Giampiero (eds.). 2018. *Atmosphere / Atmospheres: Testing a New Paradigm*. Atmospheric Spaces, 3. Milano and Udine: Mimesis International.

Gropius, Walter. 1962. *Scope of Total Architecture* (1937). New York, NY: Collier Books.

Gruppuso, Paolo. 2018. "Vapours in the Sphere: Malaria, Atmosphere and Landscape in Wet Lands of Agro Pontino, Italy." In S. Asu Schroer and S.B. Schmitt (eds.), 2018, 45–60.

Gumbrecht, Hans U. 2012. *Atmosphere, Mood, Stimmung: On a Hidden Potential of Literature* (2011). Trans. by E. Butler. Stanford, CA: Stanford University Press (SUP).

Harries, Karsten. 1983. "Thoughts on a Non-Arbitrary Architecture." *Perspecta. The Yale Architectural Journal* 20: 9–20.

Hasegawa, Yūko. 2005. *Kazuyo Sejima + Ryūe Nishizawa: SANAA*. Milano: Mondadori Electa.

Hasse, Jürgen. 1994. *Erlebnisräume: Vom Spaß zur Erfahrung*. Wien: Passagen.

Hasse, Jürgen. 2012. *Atmosphären der Stadt: Aufgespürte Räume*. Berlin: Jovis.

Hasse, Jürgen. 2014. "Atmospheres as Expression of Medial Power: Understanding Atmospheres in Urban Governance and Under Self-Guidance." *Lebenswelt. Aesthetics and Philosophy of Experience* 4 (Immagini della mente: Il desiderio), 1: 214–229. DOI: 10.13130/2240-9599/4201.

Hauskeller, Michael. 1995. *Atmosphären erleben: Philosophische Untersuchungen zur Sinneswahrnehmung*. Berlin: Akademie Verlag.

Havik, Klaske. 2019. "TerriStories: Literary Tools for Capturing Atmosphere in Architectural Pedagogy." *Ambiances. International Journal of Sensory Environment, Architecture and Urban Space* 5 (Phenomenographies: Describing Urban and Architectural Atmospheres): n.p. DOI: 10.4000/ambiances.2787.

Havik, Klaske, and Tielens, Gus. 2013a. "Concentrated Confidence: A Visit to Peter Zumthor / Geconcentreerd vertrouwen: Een bezoek aan Peter Zumthor." *OASE. Journal for Architecture / Tijdschrift voor architectuur* 91 (Building Atmosphere / Sfeer bouwen): 59–82.

Havik, Klaske, and Tielens, Gus. 2013b. "Atmosphere, Compassion and Embodied Experience: A Conversation about Atmosphere with Juhani Pallasmaa / Sfeer, mededogen en belichaamde ervaring: Een gesprek over sfeer met Juhani Pallasmaa." *OASE. Journal for Architecture / Tijdschrift voor architectuur* 91 (Building Atmosphere / Sfeer bouwen): 33–52.

Hays, K. Michael (ed.). 2008. *Buckminster Fuller: Starting with the Universe*. New York, NY: Whitney Museum of American Art — New Haven, CT and London: Yale University Press (YUP).

Heidegger, Martin. 1962. *Being and Time* (1927). Trans. by J. Macquarrie and E. Robinson. Oxford: Basil Blackwell.

Heidegger, Martin. 1975. "The Thing." In *Poetry, Language, Thought* (1971), trans. by A. Hofstadter, 163–186. New York, NY: Harper and Row.

Heyes, Cecilia, and Catmur, Caroline. 2021. "What Happened to Mirror Neurons?" *Perspectives On Psychological Science* 17, 1: 153–168. DOI: 10.1177/1745691621990638.

Hickok, Gregory. 2014. *The Myth of Mirror Neurons: The Real Neuroscience of Communication and Cognition*. New York, NY and London: W.W. Norton.

Holl, Steven, Pallasmaa, Juhani, and Pérez-Gómez, Alberto. 1994. "Questions of Perception: Phenomenology of Architecture." *A+u. Architecture and Urbanism*, special issue.

Höök, Kristina. 2018. *Designing with the Body: Somaesthetic Interaction Design*. Design Thinking, Design Theory, 15. Cambridge, MA and London: The MIT Press.

Hutmacher, Fabian. 2019. "Why Is There So Much More Research on Vision Than on Any Other Sensory Modality?" *Frontiers in Psychology* 10: 2246, 1–12. DOI: 10.3389/fpsyg.2019.02246.

Iacoboni, Marco, Molnar-Szakacs, Istvan, Gallese, Vittorio, Buccino, Giovanni, Mazziotta, John C., and Rizzolatti, Giacomo. 2005. "Grasping the Intentions of Others with One's Own Mirror Neuron System." *PLOS Biology* 3, 3: e79, 529–535. DOI: 10.1371/journal.pbio.0030079.

Imrie, Rob. 2003. "Architects' Conceptions of the Human Body." *Environment and Planning D: Society and Space* 21, 1: 47–65. DOI: 10.1068/d271t.

Ingold, Tim. 2011. *Being Alive: Essays on Movement, Knowledge and Description*. Abingdon and New York, NY: Routledge.

Ingold, Tim. 2012. "The Atmosphere." *Chiasmi International* 14 (Merleau-Ponty: Science, Images, Events): 75–87. DOI: 10.5840/chiasmi20121410.

Ingold, Tim. 2015. *The Life of Lines*. Abingdon and New York, NY: Routledge.

Ingold, Tim. 2016. "Lighting Up the Atmosphere." In *Elements of Architecture: Assembling Archaeology, Atmosphere and the Performance of Building Spaces*, ed. by M. Bille and T.F. Sørensen, 163–176. Archaeological Orientations, 3. Abingdon and New York, NY: Routledge.

Iran-Nejad, Asghar, and Irannejad, Auriana B. 2017. "Conceptual and Biofunctional Embodiment: A Long Story on the Transience of the Enduring Mind." *Frontiers in Psychology* 7: 1990, 1–6. DOI: 10.3389/fpsyg.2016.01990.

Jelić, Andrea. 2015. "Designing 'Pre-reflective' Architecture: Implications of Neurophenomenology for Architectural Design and Thinking." *Ambiances. International Journal of Sensory Environment, Architecture and Urban Space* 1 (Experiential Simulation): n.p. DOI: 10.4000/ambiances.535.

Jelić, Andrea, and Staničić, Aleksandar. 2020. "The Memory in Bodily and Architectural Making: Reflections from Embodied Cognitive Science." In *Affective Architectures: More-Than-Representational Geographies of Heritage*, ed. by J. Micieli-Voutsinas and A.M. Person. Critical Studies in Heritage, Emotion and Affect, 5. Abingdon and New York, NY: Routledge.

Jelić, Andrea, Tieri, Gaetano, De Matteis, Federico, Babiloni, Fabio, and Vecchiato, Giovanni. 2016. "The Enactive Approach to Architectural Experience: A Neurophysiological Perspective on Embodiment, Motivation, and Affordances." *Frontiers in Psychology* 7: 481, 1–20. DOI: 10.3389/fpsyg.2016.00481.

Johnson, Mark L. 1987. *The Body in the Mind: The Bodily Basis of Meaning, Imagination, and Reason*. Chicago, IL: The University of Chicago Press (UCP).

Johnson, Mark L. 2002. "Architecture and the Embodied Mind / Architectuur en de belichaamde geest." *OASE. Journal for Architecture / Tijdschrift voor architectuur* 58 (The Visible and the Invisible / Het zichtbare en het onzichtbare): 75–96.

Johnson, Mark L. 2015. "The Embodied Meaning of Architecture." In *Mind in Architecture: Neuroscience, Embodiment, and the Future of Design*, ed. by S. Robinson and J. Pallasmaa, 33–50. Cambridge, MA and London: The MIT Press. Stable URL: http://www.jstor.org/stable/j.ctt17kk8bm.6.

Julmi, Christian. 2017. *Situations and Atmospheres in Organizations: A (New) Phenomenology of Being-in-the-Organization* (2015). Atmospheric Spaces, 2. Milano and Udine: Mimesis International.

Kahn, Louis I. 1960. "Structure and Form." In *Voice of America Forum Architecture*, a radio lecture series on Modern American Architecture. V. Scully Jr. included this talk, retitled "Form and Design," in *Louis I. Kahn* (1962), 114–121. Makers of Contemporary Architecture. New York, NY: George Braziller.

Kahn, Louis I. 1961. "Kahn." *Perspecta. The Yale Architectural Journal* 7: 9–28. A discussion about the American Consulate in Luanda (Portuguese Angola), recorded in Kahn's Philadelphia office in February 1961. DOI: 10.2307/1566863.

Kahn, Louis I. 1969. "Silence and Light." Talk with students at the School of Architecture of the Eidgenössische Technische Hochschule (ETH), Zürich. 12 February 1969. Reprinted in *Louis I. Kahn: Writings, Lectures, Interviews* (1991), ed. by A. Latour, 234–246. New York, NY: Rizzoli International Publications.

Kahn, Louis I. 1973. "The Room, the Street and Human Agreement." *A+u. Architecture and Urbanism* 3, 1 (Louis I. Kahn: Silence and Light): 6–22. Reprinted in *Louis I. Kahn: Writings, Lectures, Interviews* (1991), ed. by A. Latour, 263–269. New York, NY: Rizzoli International Publications.

Kakuzō, Okakura. 1906. *The Book of Tea*. New York, NY: Duffield.

Kandel, Eric R., Schwartz, James H., and Jessell, Thomas M. (eds.). 2000. *Principles of Neural Science* (1981). 4th edn. New York, NY: McGraw-Hill.

Kandel, Eric R., Schwartz, James H., Jessell, Thomas M., Siegelbaum, Steven A., and Hudspeth, A. James (eds.). 2013. *Principles of Neural Science* (1981). 5th edn. New York, NY: McGraw-Hill.

Kandel, Eric R., Koester, John D., Mack, Sarah H., and Siegelbaum, Steven A. (eds.). 2021. *Principles of Neural Science* (1981). 6th edn. New York, NY: McGraw-Hill.

Karandinou, Anastasia. 2013. *No Matter: Theories and Practices of the Ephemeral in Architecture*. Studies in Architecture, 8. Farnham and Burlington, VT: Ashgate.

Karjalainen, Timo P. 2015. "On Topobiography: Or, How to Write One's Place." *Nordia Geographical Publications* 44, 4 (NGP Yearbook 2015: Geographies of Regions, Borders and Identity): 101–107.

Kaufmann, Edgar, and Raeburn, Ben (eds.). 1960. *Frank Lloyd Wright: Writings and Buildings*. A Meridian Book. New York, NY: New American Library.

Kazig, Rainer. 2016. "Presentation of Hermann Schmitz' paper, 'Atmospheric Spaces.'" *Ambiances. International Journal of Sensory Environment, Architecture and Urban Space*, Rediscovering: n.p. DOI: 10.4000/ambiances.709.

Kiesler, Frederick. 1949. "Pseudo-Functionalism in Modern Architecture." *Partisan Review* 16, 7: 733–742.

Kleinginna, Paul R., and Kleinginna, Anne M. 1981. "A Categorized List of Emotion Definitions, with Suggestions for a Consensual Definition." *Motivation and Emotion* 5, 4: 345–379. DOI: 10.1007/BF00992553.

Knabb, Ken (ed.). 2006. *Situationist International Anthology* (1981). Rev. and exp. edn. Berkeley, CA: Bureau of Public Secrets.

Koolhaas, Rem. 1985. "Imagining Nothingness." In *S,M,L,XL* (1995), ed. by OMA, R. Koolhaas, and B. Mau, 198–203. New York. NY: The Monacelli Press.

Koolhaas, Rem, AMO, Harvard Graduate School of Design, Boom, Irma, Trüby, Stephan, Di Robilant, Manfredo, and Westcott, James (eds.). *Elements: A Series of 15 Books Accompanying the Exhibition "Elements of Architecture" at the 2014 Venice Architecture Biennale*. Venezia: Marsilio.

Koss, Juliet. 2006. "On the Limits of Empathy." *The Art Bulletin* 88, 1: 139–157. Stable URL: https://www.jstor.org/stable/25067229.

Kotler, Philip. 1973. "Atmospherics as a Marketing Tool." *Journal of Retailing* 49: 48–64.

Krebs, Angelika. 2014. "Why Landscape Beauty Matters." *Land* 3, 4: 1251–1269. DOI:10.3390/land3041251.

Kries, Mateo, Eisenbrand, Jochen, and von Moos, Stanislaus. 2013. *Louis Kahn: The Power of Architecture*. Weil am Rhein: Vitra Design Museum.

Küller, Rikard, Ballal, Seifeddin, Laike, Thorbjörn, Mikellides, Byron, and Tonello, Graciela. 2006. "The Impact of Light and Colour on Psychological Mood: A Cross-Cultural Study of Indoor Work Environments." *Ergonomics. The Official Journal of the Chartered Institute of Ergonomics and Human Factors* 49, 14: 1496–1507. DOI: 10.1080/00140130600858142.

La Cecla, Franco. 2020. *Against Urbanism* (2014). Trans. by M. O'Mahony. San Francisco, CA: The Green Arcade — Oakland, CA: PM Press.

Labs-Ehlert, Brigitte. 2005. "Conversing with Beauty." Preface to P. Zumthor, 2006, 6–9.

Laing, Ronald D. 1967. *The Politics of Experience and The Bird of Paradise*. Middlesex: Penguin Books.

Lanzoni, Susan. 2018. *Empathy: A History*. New Haven, CT and London: Yale University Press (YUP).

Latour, Bruno. 2003. "Atmosphère, Atmosphère." In *Olafur Eliasson: The Weather Project* (exhibition catalogue), ed. by S. May, 29–41. London: Tate Publishing.

Le Corbusier. 1929. "The Pack-Donkey's Way and Man's Way." In *The City of To-morrow and its Planning* (1924), trans. by F. Etchells. London: John Rodker. Reprinted in *The Urban Design Reader* (2013), 2nd edn, ed. by M. Larice and E. Macdonald, 90–99. Urban Reader Series. Abingdon and New York, NY: Routledge.

Le Corbusier. 1931. *Towards a New Architecture* (1923). Trans. by F. Etchells. London: John Rodker.

Le Corbusier. 1948. "Ineffable Space" (1946). In *New World of Space*, 7–9. New York, NY: Reynal and Hitchcock — Boston, MA: The Institute of Contemporary Art.

Le Corbusier. 1955. *Le Poème de l'Angle Droit*. Paris: Éditions Tériade.

Le Corbusier. 2015. *Precisions on the Present State of Architecture and City Planning: Reprint of the Original American Edition* (1991). Zürich: Park Books — Paris: Fondation Le Corbusier. This work originally appeared in French under the title *Précisions sur un état present de l'architecture et de l'urbanisme* (1930). Paris: G. Crès et Cie.

Leatherbarrow, David. 2015. "Atmospheric Conditions." In *Phenomenologies of the City: Studies in the History and Philosophy of Architecture*, ed. by H. Steiner and M. Sternberg, 85–100. Studies in Architecture, 5. Abingdon and New York, NY: Routledge.

Legrenzi, Paolo, and Umiltà, Carlo. 2011. *Neuromania: On the Limits of Brain Science* (2009). Trans. by F. Anderson. New York, NY: Oxford University Press (OUP).

Leiberg, Susanne, and Anders, Silke. 2006. "The Multiple Facets of Empathy: A Survey of Theory and Evidence." *Progress in Brain Research* 156: 419–440. DOI: 10.1016/S0079-6123(06)56023-6.

Leitner, Bernhard, and Conrads, Ulrich. 1985. "Der hörbare Raum: Erfahrungen und Mutmaßungen. Gesprächsnotizen von Bernhard Leitner und Ulrich Conrads / Acoustic Space: Experiences and Conjectures. A Conversation between Bernhard Leitner and Ulrich Conrads." *Daidalos. Architektur Kunst Kultur / Architecture Art Culture* 17 (Der hörbare Raum / The Audible Space): 28–45.

Levin, David M. (ed.). 1993. *Modernity and the Hegemony of Vision*. Berkeley, CA, Los Angeles, CA, and London: University of California (UC) Press.

Lewin, Kurt. 1938. *The Conceptual Representation and the Measurement of Psychological Forces*. Durham, NC: Duke University Press (DUP).

Lipps, Theodor. 1897. *Raumästhetik und geometrisch-optischen Täuschungen*. Leipzig: Johann Ambrosius Barth.

Lipps, Theodor. 1906. "Einfühlung und ästhetischer Genuß." *Die Zukunft* 54: 110–114.

Lo Ricco, Gabriella, and Micheli, Silvia. 2003. *Lo spettacolo dell'architettura: Profilo dell'archistar®*. Milano: Bruno Mondadori.

Lobell, John. 1979. *Between Silence and Light: Spirit in the Architecture of Louis I. Kahn*. Boston, MA: Shambhala Publications.

Luhmann, Niklas. 2000. *Art as a Social System* (1995). Trans. by E.M. Knodt. Stanford, CA: Stanford University Press (SUP).

Lupton, Ellen, and Lipps, Andrea. 2018. *The Senses: Design Beyond Vision*. Hudson, NY: Princeton Architectural Press — New York, NY: Cooper Hewitt, Smithsonian Design Museum.

Mallgrave, Harry F. 2010. *The Architect's Brain: Neuroscience, Creativity, and Architecture*. Chichester: Wiley-Blackwell.

Mallgrave, Harry F. 2013. *Architecture and Embodiment: The Implications of the New Sciences and Humanities for Design*. Abingdon and New York, NY: Routledge.

Mallgrave, Harry F. 2015a. "Enculturation, Sociality, and the Built Environment." In P. Tidwell (ed.), 2015, 20–41.

Mallgrave, Harry F. 2015b. "Embodiment and Enculturation: The Future of Architectural Design." *Frontiers in Psychology* 6: 1398, 1–5. DOI: 10.3389/fpsyg.2015.01398.

Mallgrave, Harry F. 2018. *From Object to Experience: The New Culture of Architectural Design*. London and New York, NY: Bloomsbury.

Mallgrave, Harry F., and Gepshtein, Sergei. 2021. "The Interface of Two Cultures." *Intertwining* 3 (Weaving Body Context): 48–73.

Mallgrave, Harry F., and Ikonomou, Eleftherios (eds. and trans.). 1994. *Empathy, Form, and Space: Problems in German Aesthetics. 1873–1893*. Texts and Documents Series. Santa Monica, CA: Getty Center for the History of Art and the Humanities.

Martin, Craig. 2015. "The Invention of Atmosphere." *Studies in History and Philosophy of Science* 52: 44–54. DOI: 10.1016/j.shpsa.2015.05.007.

Martin, Daryl, Nettleton, Sarah, and Buse, Christina. 2019. "Affecting Care: Maggie's Centres and the Orchestration of Architectural Atmospheres." *Social Science and Medicine* 240: 112563, 1–8. DOI: 10.1016/j.socscimed.2019.112563.

Marton, Ference. 1981. "Phenomenography: Describing Conceptions of the World around Us." *Instructional Science* 10, 2: 177–200. Stable URL: https://www.jstor.org/stable/23368358.

McCarter, Robert. 2005. *Louis I Kahn*. London and New York, NY: Phaidon.

McGilchrist, Iain. 2019. *The Master and His Emissary: The Divided Brain and the Making of the Western World* (2009). 2rd edn, expanded version. New Haven, CT and London: Yale University Press (YUP).

McLuhan, Marshall. 1964. *Understanding Media: The Extensions of Man*. 2nd edn. A Mentor Book. New York, NY: New American Library.

Melandri, Enzo. 1968. *La linea e il circolo: Studio logico-filosofico sull'analogia*. Bologna: Il Mulino.

Merleau-Ponty, Maurice. 1964. "Eye and Mind" (1961). In *The Primacy of Perception: And Other Essays on Phenomenological Psychology, the Philosophy of Art, History and Politics*. Ed. by J.M. Edie. Trans. by C. Dallery, 159–190. Evanston, IL: Northwestern University Press (NUP).

Merleau-Ponty, Maurice. 1968. *The Visible and the Invisible* (1964). Ed. By C. Lefort. Trans. by A. Lingis. Studies in Phenomenology and Existential Philosophy. Evanston, IL: Northwestern University Press (NUP).

Merleau-Ponty, Maurice. 2002. *Phenomenology of Perception* (1945). Trans. by C. Smith. London and New York, NY: Routledge.

Mies van der Rohe, Ludwig. 1991. "Office Building" (1923). In *The Artless Word: Mies van der Rohe on the Building Art*, ed. by F. Neumeyer, 241. Cambridge, MA and London: The MIT Press.

Mostafavi, Armin. 2021. "Architecture, Biometrics, and Virtual Environments Triangulation: A Research Review." *Architectural Science Review*, n.n.: 1–18. DOI: 10.1080/00038628.2021.2008300.

Moussavi, Farshid, and Kubo, Michael (eds.). 2008. *The Function of Ornament*. Barcelona and New York, NY: Actar — Cambridge, MA: Harvard University, Graduate School of Design (GSD).

Nagel, Thomas. 1974. "What Is It Like to Be a Bat?" *The Philosophical Review* 83, 4: 435–450. DOI: 10.2307/2183914.

Neisser, Ulrich G. 1967. *Cognitive Psychology*. New York, NY: Appleton-Century-Crofts (ACC).

Neutra, Richard J. 1954. *Survival Through Design*. New York, NY: Oxford University Press (OUP).

Newen, Albert, De Bruin, Leon, and Gallagher, Shaun (eds.). 2018. *The Oxford Handbook of 4E Cognition*. New York, NY: Oxford University Press (OUP).

Newman, Winifred E. 2018. "Counter Re-formations of Embodiment." *Log* 42 (Disorienting Phenomenology): 165–169. Stable URL: https://www.jstor.org/stable/44840738.

Noever, Peter (ed.). 2001. *James Turrell: The Other Horizon*. Berlin: Hatje Cantz.

Norberg-Schulz, Christian. 1971. *Existence, Space and Architecture*. London: Studio Vista.

Norberg-Schulz, Christian. 1979. *Genius Loci: Towards a Phenomenology of Architecture*. New York, NY: Rizzoli International Publications.

Norberg-Schulz, Christian. 1980. *Louis I. Kahn: Idea e Immagine*. Trans. by A.M. De Dominicis. Roma: Officina Edizioni.

Nowak, Magdalena. 2011. "The Complicated History of *Einfühlung*." *Argument. Biannual Philosophical Journal* 1, 2: 301–326.

Ohrstedt, Pernilla, and Isaacs, Hayley. 2010. *Hylozoic Ground: Liminal Responsive Architecture. Philip Beesley*. Cambridge: Riverside Architectural Press.

Oliva, Stefano. 2015. "Il sentimento è un'atmosfera? Il paradigma musicale del 'terzo' Wittgenstein." *De Musica* 19: 227–246.

O'Neill, Máire E. 2001. "Corporeal Experience: A Haptic Way of Knowing." *Journal of Architectural Education* 55, 1: 3–12. Stable URL: https://www.jstor.org/stable/1425670.

Osler, Lucy, and Szanto, Thomas. 2021. "Political Emotions and Political Atmospheres." In *Shared Emotions and Atmospheres*, ed. by D. Trigg, 162–188. Ambiances, Atmospheres and Sensory Experiences of Spaces, 9. Abingdon and New York, NY: Routledge.

Ottolini, Gianni. 2010. *La stanza*. Cinisello Balsamo: Silvana Editoriale.

Pallasmaa, Juhani. 1994. "An Architecture of the Seven Senses." In S. Holl, J. Pallasmaa, and A. Pérez-Gómez, (eds.), 1994, 27–37.

Pallasmaa, Juhani. 1998. "Logic of the Image." *The Journal of Architecture* 3, 4: 289–299. DOI: 10.1080/136023698374080.

Pallasmaa, Juhani. 2000. "Hapticity and Time: Notes on Fragile Architecture." *The Architectural Review* 1239, vol. CCVII, 5 (Materiality): 78–84.

Pallasmaa, Juhani. 2002. "Lived Space: Embodied Experience and Sensory Thought / Geleefde ruimte: Belichaamde ervaring en zintuiglijk denken." *OASE. Journal for Architecture / Tijdschrift voor architectuur* 58 (The Visible and the Invisible / Het zichtbare en het onzichtbare): 13–34.

Pallasmaa, Juhani. 2009a. *The Thinking Hand: Existential and Embodied Wisdom in Architecture*. Architectural Design Primers. Chichester: Wiley.

Pallasmaa, Juhani. 2009b. "Space, Place, Memory, and Imagination: The Temporal Dimension of Existential Space." In *Spatial Recall: Memory in Architecture and Landscape*, ed. by M. Treib, 16–41. Abingdon and New York, NY: Routledge.

Pallasmaa, Juhani. 2011a. "Selfhood and the World: Lived Space, Vision and Hapticity." In *Senses and the City: An Interdisciplinary Approach to Urban Sensescapes*, ed. by M. Diaconu, E. Heuberger, R. Mateus-Berr, and L.M. Vosicky, 49–62. Wien and Münster: Lit Verlag.

Pallasmaa, Juhani. 2011b. *The Embodied Image: Imagination and Imagery in Architecture*. Architectural Design Primers. Chichester: Wiley.

Pallasmaa, Juhani. 2012a. *The Eyes of the Skin: Architecture and the Senses* (1996). 3rd edn. Chichester: Wiley.

Pallasmaa, Juhani. 2012b. "The Existential Image: Lived Space in Cinema and Architecture." *Phainomenon. Journal of Phenomenological Philosophy* 25: 157–174.

Pallasmaa, Juhani. 2013. "Orchestrating Architecture: Atmosphere in Frank Lloyd Wright's Buildings / Het orkestreren van architectuur: Sfeer in de gebouwen van Frank Lloyd Wright." *OASE. Journal for Architecture / Tijdschrift voor architectuur* 91 (Building Atmosphere / Sfeer bouwen): 53–58.

Pallasmaa, Juhani. 2014a. "Space, Place and Atmosphere: Emotion and Peripherical Perception in Architectural Experience." *Lebenswelt. Aesthetics and Philosophy of Experience* 4, 1: 230–245. DOI: 10.13130/2240-9599/4202.

Pallasmaa, Juhani. 2014b. "Empathic and Embodied Imagination: Intuiting Life and Experience in Architecture." In *ANFA 2014 Conference: Presenter Abstracts*, ed. by the Academy of Neuroscience for Architecture (ANFA), 76–77. San Diego, CA: 18–20 September 2014.

Pallasmaa, Juhani. 2014c. "A Conversation on Atmosphere." With G. Böhme, T. Griffero, and J.P. Thibaud. In P. Tidwell (ed.), 2014, 67–77.

Pallasmaa, Juhani. 2015. "Body, Mind, and Imagination: The Mental Essence of Architecture." In *Mind in Architecture: Neuroscience, Embodiment, and the Future of Design*, ed. by S. Robinson and J. Pallasmaa, 51–74. Cambridge, MA and London: The MIT Press. Stable URL: http://www.jstor.org/stable/j.ctt17kk8bm.7.

Pallasmaa, Juhani. 2016a. "Matter, Hapticity and Time: Material Imagination and the Voice of Matter." *Building Material* 20 (Building Material): 171–189. Stable URL: https://www.jstor.org/stable/26445108.

Pallasmaa, Juhani. 2016b. "The Sixth Sense: The Meaning of Atmosphere and Mood." *AD. Architectural Design* 86, 6 (Evoking Through Design: Contemporary Moods in Architecture): 126–133. DOI: 10.1002/ad.2121.

Pallasmaa, Juhani. 2017. "Between the Realities of Science and Art." In *Olafur Eliasson: Pentagonal Landscape* (exhibition catalogue), 46–51. Espoo: Espoo Museum of Modern Art (EMMA).

Pallasmaa, Juhani, and Zambelli, Matteo. 2020. *Inseminations: Seeds for Architectural Thought* (2011). Chichester and Hoboken, NJ: Wiley.

Papale, Paolo, Chiesi, Leonardo, Rampinini, Alessandra C., Pietrini, Pietro, and Ricciardi, Emiliano. 2016. "When Neuroscience 'Touches' Architecture: From Hapticity to a Supramodal Functioning of the Human Brain." *Frontiers in Psychology* 7: 866, 1–8. DOI: 10.3389/fpsyg.2016.00866.

Pasqualini, Isabella, and Blanke, Olaf. 2014. "The Self-Conscious Observer: Embodiment and Bodily Feelings in Architecture." In *Körperbilder in Kunst und Wissenschaft*, ed. by W.G. Schmidt, 31–58. Würzburg: Königshausen and Neumann.

Pasqualini, Isabella, Llobera, Joan, and Blanke, Olaf. 2013. "'Seeing' and 'Feeling' Architecture: How Bodily Self-Consciousness Alters Architectonic Experience and Affects the Perception of Interiors." *Frontiers in Psychology* 4: 354: 1–10. DOI: 10.3389/fpsyg.2013.00354.

Pérez Liebergesell, Natalia, Vermeersch, Peter-Willem, and Heylighen, Ann. 2019. "Through the Eyes of a Deaf Architect: Reconsidering Conventional Critiques of Vision-Centered Architecture." *The Senses and Society* 14, 1: 46–62. DOI: 10.1080/17458927.2019.1569349.

Pérez-Gómez, Alberto. 2002. "Phenomenology and Virtual Space: Alternative Tactics for Architectural Practice / Fenomenologie en virtuele ruimte: Alternatieve strategieën voor de architectuurpraktijk." *OASE. Journal for Architecture / Tijdschrift voor architectuur* 58 (The Visible and the Invisible / Het zichtbare en het onzichtbare): 35–58.

Pérez-Gómez, Alberto. 2016. *Attunement: Architectural Meaning After the Crisis of Modern Science*. Cambridge, MA and London: The MIT Press.

Peri Bader, Aya. 2015. "A Model for Everyday Experience of the Built Environment: The Embodied Perception of Architecture." *The Journal of Architecture* 20, 2: 244–267. DOI: 10.1080/13602365.2015.1026835.

Perrot, Michelle. 2018. *The Bedroom: An Intimate History* (2009). Trans. by L. Elkin. New Haven, CT and London: Yale University Press (YUP).

Pert, Candace B. 1997. *Molecules of Emotion: Why You Feel the Way You Feel*. New York, NY: Scribner.

Petitot, Jean, Varela, Francisco J., Pachoud, Bernard, and Roy, Jean-Michel. 1999. *Naturalizing Phenomenology: Issues in Contemporary Phenomenology and Cognitive Science*. Stanford, CA: Stanford University Press (SUP).

Pile, Steve. 2010. "Emotions and Affect in Recent Human Geography." *TIBG. Transactions of the Institute of British Geographers* 35, 1: 5–20. DOI: 10.1111/j.1475-5661.2009.00368.x.

Plummer, Henry. 2016. *The Experience of Architecture*. London: Thames and Hudson (T&H).

Ponti, Gio. 1960. *In Praise of Architecture* (1957). Trans. by G. Salvadori and M. Salvadori. New York, NY: F.W. Dodge Corporation.

Purves, Dale, Cabeza, Roberto, Huettel, Scott A., LaBar, Kevin S., Platt, Michael L., and Woldorff, Marty G. (eds.). 2012. *Principles of Cognitive Neuroscience* (2007). 2nd edn. New York, NY: Oxford University Press (OUP).

Purves, Dale, Augustine, George J., Fitzpatrick, David, Hall, William C., LaMantia, Anthony-Samuel, Mooney, Richard D., Platt, Michael L., and White, Leonard E. (eds.). 2018. *Neuroscience*. 6th edn. New York, NY: Oxford University Press (OUP).

Rahm, Philippe. 2009. *Architecture météorologique*. Paris: Archibooks.

Rahm, Philippe. 2015. *Météorologie des sentiments*. Paris: Les Petits Matins.

Rahm, Philippe. 2018. "Meteorology." *Domus* 1020 (Rebellion. Audacity. Courage. Daring): 106–107.

Rahm, Philippe. 2020. "Climatorium: Architect as Meteorologist / L'architetto come meteorologo." *Vesper. Journal of Architecture, Arts and Theory / Rivista di architettura, arti e teoria* 2 (Author — Matter / Materia — Autore): 24–35.

Rasmussen, Steen E. 1959. *Experiencing Architecture* (1957). Cambridge, MA and London: The MIT Press.

Rauh, Andreas. 2017. "In the Clouds: On the Vagueness of Atmospheres." *Ambiances. International Journal of Sensory Environment, Architecture and Urban Space*, Varia: n.p. DOI: 10.4000/ambiances.818.

Rauh, Andreas. 2018. *Concerning Astonishing Atmospheres: Aisthesis, Aura, and Atmospheric Portfolio*. Atmospheric Spaces, 4. Milano and Udine: Mimesis International.

Riedel, Friedlind. 2019. "Atmosphere." In *Affective Societies: Key Concepts*, ed. by J. Slaby and C. von Scheve, 85–95. Routledge Studies in Affective Societies, 5. Abingdon and New York, NY: Routledge.

Riedel, Friedlind. 2020. "Atmospheric Relations: Theorising Music and Sound as Atmosphere." In *Music as Atmosphere: Collective Feelings and Affective Sounds*, ed. by F. Riedel and J. Torvinen, 1–42. Ambiances, Atmospheres and Sensory Experiences of Spaces, 4. Abingdon and New York, NY: Routledge.

Rizzolatti, Giacomo, and Fogassi, Leonardo. 2014. "The Mirror Mechanism: Recent Findings and Perspectives." *Philosophical Transactions of the Royal Society B. Biological Sciences* 369, 1644: 20130420, 1–12. DOI: 10.1098/rstb.2013.0420.

Rizzolatti, Giacomo, Fogassi, Leonardo, and Gallese, Vittorio. 2001. "Neurophysiological Mechanisms Underlying the Understanding and Imitation of Action." *Nature Reviews Neuroscience* 2, 9: 661–670. DOI: 10.1038/35090060.

Rizzolatti, Giacomo, and Sinigaglia, Corrado. 2006. *So quel che fai: Il cervello che agisce e i neuroni specchio*. Scienza e Idee. Milano: Raffaello Cortina.

Rizzolatti, Giacomo, and Sinigaglia, Corrado. 2008. *Mirrors in the Brain: How Our Minds Share Actions and Emotions* (2006). Trans. by F. Anderson. New York, NY: Oxford University Press (OUP).

Robinson, Jenefer M. 2012. "On Being Moved by Architecture." *The Journal of Aesthetics and Art Criticism* 70, 4: 337–353. Stable URL: https://www.jstor.org/stable/43496529.

Robinson, Sarah. 2011. *Nesting: Body Dwelling Mind*. San Francisco, CA: William Stout.

Robinson, Sarah. 2021. *Architecture is a Verb*. Abingdon and New York, NY: Routledge.

Robinson, Sarah. 2022. "How 4E Cognition Changes Architectural Design Education." *Architecture, Structures and Construction*, n.n.: 1–6. DOI: 10.1007/s44150-022-00028-x.

Romano, Giovanni. 1941. "La casa di un architetto." *Domus* 163, year XIX, 7: 9–17.

Rooney, Kevin K. 2016. "Vision and the Experience of Built Environments: Two Visual Pathways of Awareness, Attention and Embodiment in Architecture." Doctoral dissertation, Kansas State University. K-State Research Exchange (K-REx): http://hdl.handle.net/2097/20597.

Rooney, Kevin K., Condia, Robert J., and Loschky, Lester C. 2017. "Focal and Ambient Processing of Built Environments: Intellectual and Atmospheric Experiences of Architecture." *Frontiers in Psychology* 8: 326, 1–20. DOI: 10.3389/fpsyg.2017.00326.

Rossi, Aldo. 1984. *The Architecture of the City* (1966). Trans. by D. Ghirardo and J. Ockman. American edn. rev. by A. Rossi and P. Eisenman. Oppositions Books Series. Cambridge, MA and London: The MIT Press.

Rykwert, Joseph. 2000. *The Seduction of Place: The City in the Twenty-First Century*. New York, NY: Pantheon Books.

Sadler, Simon. 1999. *The Situationist City*. Cambridge, MA and London: The MIT Press.

Sambonet, Guia (ed.). 1998. *James Turrell: Dipinto con la luce*. Milano: Federico Motta.

Sbriscia-Fioretti, Beatrice, Berchio, Cristina, Freedberg, David, Gallese, Vittorio, and Umiltà, Maria A. 2013. "ERP Modulation during Observation of Abstract Paintings by Franz Kline." *PLOS One* 8, 10: e75241, 1–12. DOI: 10.1371/journal.pone.0075241.

Scelsi, Valter. 2021. "Prossimità e progetto / Proximity and Project." In *Un anno di didattica: Innovazione e ricerca nella Scuola di Architettura di Genova*, 9–11; 130–131. Opera metrica, 4. Genova: Sagep editori.

Schmarsow, August. 1994. "The Essence of Architectural Creation" (1893). In H.F. Mallgrave and E. Ikonomou (eds. and trans.), 1994, 281–297.

Schmitz, Hermann. 1967. *System der Philosophie: Der leibliche Raum*, vol. III/1. Bonn: Bouvier.

Schmitz, Hermann. 2014. *Atmosphären*. Freiburg and München: Karl Alber.

Schmitz, Hermann. 2016. "Atmospheric Spaces" (2012). Trans. by M. Vince. *Ambiances. International Journal of Sensory Environment, Architecture and Urban Space*, Rediscovering: n.p. DOI: 10.4000/ambiances.711.

Schmitz, Hermann. 2019. *New Phenomenology: A Brief Introduction* (2009). Trans. by R.O. Müllan with the support from M. Bastert. Atmospheric Spaces, 6. Milano and Udine: Mimesis International.

Schönhammer, Rainer. 2018. "Atmosphere — The Life of a Place: The Psychology of Environment and Design" (2012). In *Designing Atmospheres*, ed. by J. Weidinger, 141–179. Berlin: Universitätsverlag der TU Berlin.

Schreuder, Eliane, van Erp, Jan, Toet, Alexander, and Kallen, Victor L. 2016. "Emotional Responses to Multisensory Environmental Stimuli: A Conceptual Framework and Literature Review." *SAGE Open* 6, 1: 1–19. DOI: 10.1177/2158244016630591.

Semper, Gottfried. 1989. *The Four Elements of Architecture* (1851). Trans. by H.F. Mallgrave and W. Herrmann. Cambridge and New York, NY: Cambridge University Press (CUP). Reprinted in *Reader: Tectonics in Architecture* (2018), ed. by I.W. Foged and M.F. Hvejsel, 21–46. Aalborg: Aalborg University Press.

Semper, Gottfried. 2004. *Style in the Technical and Tectonic Arts; or, Practical Aesthetics* (1860). Trans. by H.F. Mallgrave and M. Robinson. Los Angeles, CA: Getty Research Institute.

Shusterman, Richard. 1999. "Somaesthetics: A Disciplinary Proposal." *The Journal of Aesthetics and Art Criticism* 57, 3: 299–313. DOI: 10.2307/432196.

Shusterman, Richard. 2000. *Performing Live: Aesthetic Alternatives for the Ends of Art*. Ithaca, NY and London: Cornell University Press.

Shusterman, Richard. 2006. "Thinking through the Body, Educating for the Humanities: A Plea for Somaesthetics." *The Journal of Aesthetic Education* 40, 1: 1–21. Stable URL: https://www.jstor.org/stable/4140215.

Sloterdijk, Peter. 2009. *Terror from the Air* (2002). Trans. by A. Patton and S. Corcoran. Los Angeles, CA: Semiotext(e).

Sloterdijk, Peter. 2011. *Spheres. Volume I: Bubbles. Microspherology* (1998). Trans. by W. Hoban. Foreign Agents Series. Los Angeles, CA: Semiotext(e).

Sloterdijk, Peter. 2014. *Spheres. Volume II: Globes. Macrospherology* (1999). Trans. by W. Hoban. Foreign Agents Series. Los Angeles, CA: Semiotext(e).

Sloterdijk, Peter. 2016. *Spheres. Volume III: Foams. Plural Spherology* (2004). Trans. by W. Hoban. Foreign Agents Series. Los Angeles, CA: Semiotext(e).

Soentgen, Jens. 1998. *Die verdeckte Wirklichkeit: Einführung in die Neue Phänomenologie von Hermann Schmitz*. Bonn: Bouvier.

Speer, Albert. 1970. *Inside the Third Reich: Memoirs by Albert Speer* (1969). Trans. by R. Winston and C. Winston. New York, NY: The Macmillan Company.

Spence, Charles. 2020. "Senses of Place: Architectural Design for the Multisensory Mind." *Cognitive Research: Principles and Implications* 5: 46, 1–26. DOI: 10.1186/s41235-020-00243-4.
Spitzer, Leo. 1942a. "Milieu and Ambiance: An Essay in Historical Semantics." *Philosophy and Phenomenological Research* 3, 1: 1–42. DOI: 10.2307/2103127.
Spitzer, Leo. 1942b. "Milieu and Ambiance: An Essay in Historical Semantics." *Philosophy and Phenomenological Research* 3, 2: 169–218. DOI: 10.2307/2102775.
Spitzer, Leo. 1963. *Classical and Christian Ideas of World Harmony: Prolegomena to an Interpretation of the Word "Stimmung."* Ed. by A. Granville Hatcher. Baltimore, MD: The Johns Hopkins University (JHU) Press.
Stec, Barbara. 2004. "Conversazioni con Peter Zumthor / Conversations with Peter Zumthor." *Casabella* 719, year LXVIII, 2: 6–13; 90–95.
Stec, Barbara. 2020. *Sunlight, Atmosphere and Architecture* (2017). Trans. by K. Barnaś. Kraków: AFM Publishing House.
Steiner, Dietmar. 1997. "Peter Zumthor: Bagni termali, Vals, Svizzera / Thermal Bath, Vals, Switzerland." *Domus* 798: 27–35.
Ströker, Elisabeth. 1965. *Philosophische Untersuchungen zum Raum*. Frankfurt am Main: Vittorio Klostermann.
Sullivan, Louis H. 1979. "Ornament in Architecture." In *Kindergarten Chats and Other Writings* (1918), 187–190. New York, NY: Dover Publications. First published: 1892. *The Engineering Magazine* 3: 633–634.
Sumartojo, Shanti, and Pink, Sarah. 2019. *Atmospheres and the Experiential World: Theory and Methods*. Ambiances, Atmospheres and Sensory Experiences of Space, 2. Abingdon and New York, NY: Routledge.

Tanizaki, Jun'ichirō. 2001. *In Praise of Shadows* (1933). Trans. by T.J. Harper and E.G. Seidensticker. London: Vintage Books.
Tellenbach, Hubertus. 1968. *Geschmack und Atmosphäre: Medien menschlichen Elementarkontaktes*. Salzburg: Otto Müller.
Tellenbach, Hubertus. 1981. "Tasting and Smelling — Taste and Atmosphere — Atmosphere and Trust." *Journal of Phenomenological Psychology* 12, 2: 221–230. DOI: 10.1163/156916281X00254.
Thibaud, Jean-Paul. 2014a. "Installing an Atmosphere." In P. Tidwell (ed.), 2014, 49–66.
Thibaud, Jean-Paul. 2014b. "A Conversation on Atmosphere." With G. Böhme, T. Griffero, and J. Pallasmaa. In P. Tidwell (ed.), 2014, 67–77.
Thibaud, Jean-Paul. 2015. "The Backstage of Urban Ambiances: When Atmospheres Pervade Everyday Experience." *Emotion, Space and Society* 15: 39–46. DOI: 10.1016/j.emospa.2014.07.001.
Thiis-Evensen, Thomas. 1987. *Archetypes in Architecture* (1982). Trans. by R. Waaler and S. Campbell. Oslo: Universitetsforlaget AS.
Tidwell, Philip (ed.). 2013. *Architecture and Neuroscience*. Espoo: Tapio Wirkkala — Rut Bryk (TWRB) Foundation.
Tidwell, Philip (ed.). 2014. *Architecture and Atmosphere*. Espoo: Tapio Wirkkala — Rut Bryk (TWRB) Foundation.

Tidwell, Philip (ed.). 2015. *Architecture and Empathy*. Espoo: Tapio Wirkkala — Rut Bryk (TWRB) Foundation.

Titchener, Edward B. 1909. *Lectures on the Experimental Psychology of the Thought-Processes*. New York, NY: The Macmillan Company.

Tuan, Yi-Fu. 1974. *Topophilia: A Study of Environmental Perception, Attitudes, and Values*. Englewood Cliffs, NJ: Prentice-Hall.

Turley, Lou W., and Milliman, Ronald E. 2000. "Atmospheric Effects on Shopping Behavior: A Review of the Experimental Evidence." *Journal of Business Research* 49, 2: 193–211. DOI: 10.1016/S0148-2963(99)00010-7.

Umiltà, Maria A., Berchio, Cristina, Sestito, Mariateresa, Freedberg, David, and Gallese Vittorio. 2012. "Abstract Art and Cortical Motor Activation: An EEG Study." *Frontiers in Human Neuroscience* 6: 311, 1–9. DOI: 10.3389/fnhum.2012.00311.

Varela, Francisco J. 1996. "Neurophenomenology: A Methodological Remedy for the Hard Problem." *Journal of Consciousness Studies* 3, 4: 330–349.

Varela, Francisco J., Thompson, Evan, and Rosch, Eleanor. 1991. *The Embodied Mind: Cognitive Science and Human Experience*. Cambridge, MA and London: The MIT Press.

Vecchiato, Giovanni, Tieri, Gaetano, Jelić, Andrea, De Matteis, Federico, Maglione, Anton G., and Babiloni, Fabio. 2015. "Electroencephalographic Correlates of Sensorimotor Integration and Embodiment during the Appreciation of Virtual Architectural Environments." *Frontiers in Psychology* 6: 1944, 1–18. DOI: 10.3389/fpsyg.2015.01944.

Vischer, Robert. 1994. "On the Optical Sense of Form: A Contribution to Aesthetics" (1873). In H.F. Mallgrave and E. Ikonomou (eds. and trans.), 1994, 89–123.

Von Meiss, Pierre. 1990. *Elements of Architecture: From Form to Place* (1986). New York, NY: E. and F.N. Spon.

Wagenfeld, Malte. 2013. "Aesthetics of Air." Doctoral dissertation, Royal Melbourne Institute of Technology (RMIT). RMIT Research Repository: 9921861384201341.

Wagenfeld, Malte. 2015a. "The Phenomenology of Visualizing Atmosphere." *Environmental and Architectural Phenomenology* 26, 2: 9–15.

Wagenfeld, Malte. 2015b. "Perceiving Atmospheres: A Phenomenological Exploration." In *Perception in Architecture: Here and Now*, ed. by C. Perren and M. Mlecek, 118–134. Newcastle upon Tyne: Cambridge Scholars Publishing.

Ward, Dave, and Stapleton, Mog. 2012. "Es are Good: Cognition as Enacted, Embodied, Embedded, Affective and Extended." In *Consciousness in Interaction: The Role of the Natural and Social Context in Shaping Consciousness*, ed. by F. Paglieri, 89–104. Amsterdam and Philadelphia, PA: John Benjamins.

Warhol, Andy. 1975. *The Philosophy of Andy Warhol: From A to B and Back Again*. New York, NY and London: Harcourt Brace Jovanovich.

Wegerhoff, Erik. 2016. "Neue Sinnlichkeit: Postcritical Issues Regarding an Architecture of Sensuousness." *Future Anterior. Journal of Historic Preservation, History, Theory, and Criticism* 13, 2: 119–137. DOI:10.5749/futuante.13.2.0119.

Wehrle, Maren. 2020. "Being a Body and Having a Body: The Twofold Temporality of Embodied Intentionality." *Phenomenology and the Cognitive Sciences* 19: 499–521. DOI: 10.1007/s11097-019-09610-z.

Wigley, Mark. 1998a. "Die Architektur der Atmosphäre / The Architecture of Atmosphere." *Daidalos. Architektur Kunst Kultur / Architecture Art Culture* 68 (Konstruktion von Atmosphären / Constructing Atmospheres): 18–27.

Wigley, Mark (ed.). 1998b. *Constant's New Babylon: The Hyper-Architecture of Desire*. Rotterdam: Witte de With, Center for Contemporary Art — Rotterdam: 010 Publishers.

Wright, Frank Lloyd. 1954. *The Natural House*. New York, NY: Horizon Press.

Wölfflin, Heinrich. 1994. "Prolegomena to a Psychology of Architecture" (1886). In H.F. Mallgrave and E. Ikonomou (eds. and trans.), 1994, 149–190.

Worringer, Wilhelm. 1997. *Abstraction and Empathy: A Contribution to the Psychology of Style* (1908). Trans. by M. Bullock. Elephant Paperbacks edn. Chicago, IL: Ivan R. Dee.

Zevi, Bruno. 1993. *Architecture as Space: How to Look at Architecture* (1948). Ed. by J.A. Barry. Trans. by M. Gendel. New York, NY: Da Capo Press.

Zhang, Dora. 2018. "Notes on Atmosphere." *Qui Parle. Critical Humanities and Social Sciences* 27, 1: 121–155. DOI: 10.1215/10418385-4383010.

Zumthor, Peter. 1988. "A Way of Looking at Things." In *Thinking Architecture* (1998), 9–26. Basel, Berlin, and Boston, MA: Birkhäuser.

Zumthor, Peter. 1997. "Le terme di Vals: Pietra e acqua." *Casabella* 648, year LXI, 9: 56–75.

Zumthor, Peter. 1998. *Peter Zumthor Works: Buildings and Projects. 1979–1997*. Basel, Berlin, and Boston, MA: Birkhäuser.

Zumthor, Peter. 2006. *Atmospheres: Architectural Environments. Surrounding Objects*. Basel, Berlin, and Boston, MA: Birkhäuser.

Zumthor, Peter, and Hauser, Sigrid. 2007. *Peter Zumthor: Therme Vals*. Zürich: Scheidegger und Spiess.

Zumthor, Peter, and Mostafavi, Mohsen. 1996. *Thermal Bath at Vals*. Architectural Association: Exemplary Projects, 1. London: Architectural Association Publications.

MIMESIS GROUP
www.mimesis-group.com

MIMESIS INTERNATIONAL
www.mimesisinternational.com
info@mimesisinternational.com

MIMESIS EDIZIONI
www.mimesisedizioni.it
mimesis@mimesisedizioni.it

ÉDITIONS MIMÉSIS
www.editionsmimesis.fr
info@editionsmimesis.fr

MIMESIS COMMUNICATION
www.mim-c.net

MIMESIS EU
www.mim-eu.com

Printed by
Puntoweb s.r.l. – Ariccia (RM)
April 2022